ℰVERYTHING YOU EVER WANTED TO KNOW ABOUT COSMETIC SURGERY*

*BUT COULDN'T AFFORD TO ASK

Everything YOU EVER WANTED TO KNOW ABOUT COSMETIC SURGERY*

*BUT COULDN'T AFFORD TO ASK

*A Complete Look at the Latest Techniques
and Why They Are Safer and Less Expensive
by One of Today's Most Prominent
Cosmetic Surgeons*

ALAN GAYNOR, M.D.

BROADWAY BOOKS

NEW YORK

BROADWAY

Broadway Books titles may be purchased for business or promotional use or for special sales. For information, please write to: Special Markets Department, Bantam Doubleday Dell Publishing Group, Inc., 1540 Broadway, New York, NY 10036.

BROADWAY BOOKS and its logo, a letter B bisected on the diagonal, are trademarks of Broadway Books, a division of Bantam Doubleday Dell Publishing Group, Inc.

Library of Congress Cataloging-in-Publication Data
Gaynor, Alan, 1945–
Everything you ever wanted to know about cosmetic surgery but couldn't afford to ask : a complete look at the latest techniques and why they are safer and less expensive / Alan Gaynor. — 1st ed.
p.   cm.
Includes bibliographical references and index.
ISBN 0-7679-0171-1 (hardcover)
1. Surgery, Plastic—Popular works. I. Title.
RD119.G37   1998
617.9'5—dc21   97-48838
                                          CIP

FIRST EDITION

Designed by Chris Welch

98 99 00 01 02 10 9 8 7 6 5 4 3 2 1

FOR CATHERINE GAYNOR–

VISIONARY, PARTNER, FRIEND, WIFE

CONTENTS

PART II: THE PROCEDURES

Foreword

✳

WHO IS DR. ALAN GAYNOR AND WHY SHOULD YOU READ HIS BOOK?

BY DR. DOUGLAS R. ZUSMAN

Codirector of Cardiac Surgery, Hoag Hospital,
Newport Beach, California

I first met Alan Gaynor when we were at medical school to- gether which, hard as it is for me to believe (or even to say!), was more than twenty-six years ago. We became godfathers to each other's children and the best of friends (even though he went off to cosmetic surgery while I went off to cardiac), and I know that after reading this book, you'll see soon enough why I think he's just the greatest guy in every way, both as a doctor and as a human being.

Alan was extremely gifted right from the get-go, entering Juilliard music school at the age of five and being taught by the same instructors who trained Van Cliburn. He played with the New York Philharmonic under Leonard Bernstein (appearing at Carnegie Hall at age eight) and would've had a tremendous ca- reer as a pianist, except that the desire to be a doctor called out to him. Alan switched to medicine, going from Dartmouth and Columbia to Yale Medical School, which is where we met.

At one point, while interning at Yale, Alan started getting

fevers, losing weight, and feeling exhausted all the time, but he just kept right on working. Since part of medical education involves practicing on one another, he was given a physical and, as part of his own studies, he was asked to diagnose a series of X-rays. He came to one set and exclaimed that he was sure this patient must have TB. He was told that the tuberculosis diagnosis was correct, and that he was looking at his own X-rays. Alan had to take several months off and go on a regimen of drugs, but he bounced right back to finish his studies. He even won the Lange Medical Publications Award for outstanding achievement as a medical student.

One of the things I love about Alan is how, as a doctor, he's always up on the latest in his field, because he has to *know* what is the best technique and procedure for getting the job done. He heard about liposuction, liposculpture, and the carbon dioxide laser, to name three examples, and flew over to France and down to Brazil to watch the inventors use these techniques firsthand. He was deeply impressed with what these innovations could achieve and became one of the first doctors to do these surgeries in America. He then went on to refine the technique and invent the Gaynor Cannula: a small, blunt needle that allows you to liposculpt by hand with a great deal of control and much less bruising than the machine-controlled liposuction that's in general use. Since dramatic changes are happening all the time in the field of cosmetic surgery, it's crucial to have someone completely informed about the latest innovations. Over half the work done at the Alan Gaynor Aesthetic Surgery Center uses techniques that have been invented during the past five years—some by Alan himself.

Dr. Gaynor has gotten just about every commendation a practicing doctor can get, including being a Fellow of the American Academy of Cosmetic Surgery and the American Society of Dermatological Surgery, as well as a Diplomate of the American Board of Dermatology. But if you really want immediate proof of Alan's high standing in the medical community, just take a look at who wrote this book's Afterword—none other than the godfather of cosmetic surgery and inventor of the facelift himself, Dr. Ivo Pitanguy. Pitanguy's contribution to this book shows the importance of what Alan is doing and makes a statement about the need for this type of clear information. It's crucial for patients to educate themselves as much as possible before making a decision on whether to have cosmetic surgery.

Alan's an outstanding physician, but he's also a tremendously easy person to like, with a great sense of humor and an ability to instantly make people feel relaxed and at ease. I feel honored that he asked me to write the foreword to his book, and I think it's terrific that one of the best cosmetic surgeons of our day is taking the time to explain to the lay consumer the ins and outs of his specialty. You're in for a fine education, but also for some fun along the way.

ACKNOWLEDGMENTS

A great thanks to:

Beth Gaynor, whose research, writing, and organizational skills were invaluable in the "When Vanity Is Not a Sin" chapter;

the professional members of the literary world who shepherded me along the way: Fred Hill, Bill Shinker, Lauren Marino, Craig Nelson, Irene Moore, Kati Steele;

my staff, second to none in cosmetic surgery: Telma Di Domenico, Paula Oberg, Magda Rodrigues, Cristina Santana, Eleuza Zusa;

Richard G. Glogau, M.D., San Francisco dermatologist, for making his medical library available and taking too many calls from me for additional research;

Evelyne Cohen, R.N., who was there at the beginning of liposuction and has always been there for me; and

Sterling Baker, M.D., James Romano, M.D., and Dave McDaniels, M.D.

Additionally, I want to thank many of the doctors who have helped me these last twenty-five years, without whom I could never have become the cosmetic surgeon I am today:

hair transplant	O'Tar Norwood, M.D., dermatologist, U.S.A.
facelift	Alberto Hodara, M.D., plastic surgeon, Brazil Thomas Roberts, M.D., plastic surgeon, U.S.A.
dermabrasion	John Yarborough, M.D., dermatologist, U.S.A.
liposuction	Yves Gerard Illouz, M.D., surgeon, France Pierre Fournier, M.D., plastic surgeon, France Alberto Hodara, M.D., plastic surgeon, Brazil Jacques Ohana, M.D., plastic surgeon, France
liposculpture; fat transfer	Luiz Toledo, M.D., plastic surgeon, Brazil
neck tightening	Luiz Toledo, M.D., plastic surgeon, Brazil
laser skin resurfacing	Larry David, M.D., dermatologist, U.S.A. Cynthia Weinstein, M.D., dermatologist, Australia Thomas Roberts, M.D., plastic surgeon, U.S.A.

laser eyelid lift

Sterling Baker, M.D.,
ophthalmologist, U.S.A.
Larry David, M.D.,
dermatologist, U.S.A.
Thomas Roberts, M.D.,
plastic surgeon, U.S.A.

browlift

William Beeson, M.D.,
ear, nose, and throat specialist, U.S.A.
Alberto Hodara, M.D.,
plastic surgeon, Brazil
Greg Keller, M.D.,
ear, nose, and throat specialist, U.S.A.
Thomas Roberts, M.D.,
plastic surgeon, U.S.A.

Everything
YOU EVER WANTED
TO KNOW ABOUT
COSMETIC SURGERY*

*BUT COULDN'T AFFORD TO ASK

Introduction

TODAY'S REVOLUTION IN COSMETIC SURGERY

Are you bothered by something about your appearance? Heavy thighs, a droopy face, lines between your eyebrows that make you look angry all the time? Do you feel fresher and younger on the inside than you look on the outside? And, most important of all, how long have you been putting up with these feelings, and when are you going to do something about them?

Today, more people than ever before have decided that it's time to do something about making their outer appearance fit their inner life. In this decade, there's been a huge increase in cosmetic surgery, with liposuction alone performed on almost 200,000 Americans a year—one-fifth of whom are men. That fact shouldn't come as a surprise if you think about our demographics since, in the 1990s, one American will turn fifty every seven seconds. Can't you just imagine that giant group of aging baby boomers looking in the mirror, seeing their sags and wrinkles, and thinking, as never before, about turning back the clock?

Another key factor in today's rise of cosmetic surgery is the wrenching changes that have occurred in the workplace over the past fifteen years. *The New York Times* ran a special series of articles in 1996, now published as a book, *The Downsizing of America,* which says: "The staggering waves of layoffs that began washing over the country in the late 1970s as corporations merged, downsized, and re-engineered had failed to retreat. And those waves seemed to be crashing over an ever-widening spectrum of Americans—no longer strictly the much-battered blue-collar worker, but increasingly the once-impervious, highly educated middle- and upper-class managers and professionals, people who never thought they would face want." Every week I hear stories from patients who have lost their jobs or are in danger of losing their jobs or have been denied advancement, all because of their age.

Last year I had a patient who had just lost a high-paying sales job in computers in Silicon Valley. Of course, no one mentioned his appearance or age as a factor, but he was certain this was the reason for getting laid off. I did an upper and lower eyelid lift, a mini-facelift, and laser skin resurfacing to erase his deep crow's feet. During recovery, he organized his resume and, several weeks later, started looking for a new job. In less than two months he found a position that paid better than the job he'd lost. He told me the story of one particular sales meeting at the new company where people actually commented on his youthful appearance and thought him to be five to ten years younger than he really was.

Another woman told me how she had applied for years to get a promotion in a trucking company in Arizona and was told that she lacked the skills required for the more responsible, higher-paying job. She came to California, had similar surgery, went back to Arizona, and was offered the job she had been denied without even asking for it.

A very similar story happened to another of my patients, a dynamic woman named Tonya Hayes. She recalled:

I worked in mergers and acquisitions, and it was a big job—putting together million-dollar deals and flying to New York and across the state. When the bank closed our department, I was only thirty-six years old, and I was sure that, with my track record, it'd be no problem getting a new job. Boy, was I wrong; a whole year went by and I was still unemployed. Finally I got hold of one of the interviewers who'd turned me down on the phone and I said, "Just what is it? You know I'm as overqualified for this spot as you can get," and he actually told me, "Well Tonya, we're just looking for someone younger."

So I went to Alan for a consultation and we decided on doing both upper and lower eyelids and to fill in some wrinkles. I was very satisfied with the results. Afterward, I looked a lot fresher, attractive, and sophisticated—a woman who has it all. And right away I got a new job and made such a hit out of it that now I get feelers from marketing departments at other companies all the time.

After all I've been through, I absolutely believe in cosmetic surgery, because it allows you to be the very best you can be. No one can achieve perfection, but you know that once you've achieved the best you can, you then stop trying to be perfect.

Did cosmetic surgery actually make Tonya and these others better qualified for their jobs? Of course not. They were highly qualified in the first place. What was blocking their advancement was the perception that, because they were older looking, they were not good candidates. In the ever more competitive arena of the workplace, looking as good as possible can remove an often secret barrier to success.

If you could have the one part of your physical body that you don't like changed for the better, how would it affect your attitude about yourself? There's a lot more to aesthetic surgery than just what it can do for you on the job. The improvement in self-esteem, confidence, and outlook can be so great as to last a lifetime.

My operations director (who supervises the operating rooms), Magda Rodrigues, has noticed the extraordinary and dramatic changes in self-image that occur with so many of my patients after even the most minor work has been done—how common it is for someone to also get a new wardrobe, new hairstyle, new makeup look after their cosmetic surgery—to completely change their life. Successful cosmetic surgery can give you a powerful boost in your attitude toward yourself—the kind of self-confidence that makes anyone more attractive than simply changing the shape of their nose or tucking their waistline ever could.

Another factor in cosmetic surgery's growing popularity is the rapid advance in new techniques that have tremendously reduced the invasiveness, risk, recovery time, and visibility of the surgeries themselves:

• The neck microsuction procedure you will read about later in the book can correct "turkey necks" in men and women of any age without any skin removal or stitching, and it leaves no visible scar. People can go back to work in one or two days.

• Carbon dioxide laser skin resurfacing has replaced the far riskier and less controllable TCA and Phenol peels to correct wrinkles and scars with much more predictable and reliable healing. The same laser instrument has revolutionized eyelid surgery to correct drooping upper lids and puffy lower bags without changing the overall shape of the eyes.

• Hair is now transplanted one or two hairs at a time to yield a completely natural appearance, avoiding the unnatural, pluggy, picket-fence look so common years ago.

• Liposculpture, pioneered by Dr. Luiz Toledo of São Paulo, Brazil, removes unwanted fat bulges more delicately than before, outlines muscle groups in the stomach and legs to produce a great athletic look, and can tighten loose skin without having to actually remove it on areas such as the belly.

Were it not for these new, safer, less visible, more natural advances in cosmetic surgery techniques, many of the procedures that I and thousands of my patients have gotten would have been unacceptable to us.

Another change in the new cosmetic surgery of today is that so many of our latest techniques are small and affordable. In fact, in many instances, cosmetic surgery is one of the few medical specialties where the average bill has gone *down*. You can, of course, have a massive, Hollywood-style facelift, but (and it's a *big* but) you can also undergo small procedures to specifically fix what you uniquely need to have done, without the trauma and expense of major surgery. A mini-facelift or mini-browlift can fix the specific area you need to have done without the massive surgery of a full lift—and without the windswept "pulled" look you're so used to seeing at Oscar time. If you have a little extra fat in the hips, legs, or buttocks, and you don't like the wrinkles in your face, the new fat transfer technique lets you "plump up" the wrinkle and reshape your lower body all in one step.

To understand all the dramatic revolutions that have made my job what it is today, just consider the changes that have taken place over the past decade in what is now America's favorite cosmetic surgery: liposuction. Introduced in 1977, lipo used to be a major trauma, accompanied by a major expense. But that's all changed:

1970s liposuction	1990s liposuction
up to one-week hospital stay	home after two five-hour stays in an outpatient facility
heavy bruising and swelling	less bruising and swelling
heavy blood loss with removed fat	blood loss with removed fat 50 percent less than before
only possible to remove small amounts of fat because of tissue trauma	larger amounts of fat can be removed safely from carefully selected people
general anesthesia usually needed	general anesthesia almost never needed

bed rest needed	bed rest almost never necessary; people up and walking around the next day
two to four weeks of recovery	two to five days of recovery
large incisions needed	very small incisions needed
could only be done in young people with good skin tone	can be done on people of almost any age; loose skin can now be tightened without having to actually remove it
easily could cost more than $20,000 (in 1970s dollars)!	average cost for one area $3,000 to $5,000; full body $8,000 to $12,000

New techniques, new attitudes, less trauma, less expense: This is today's revolution in cosmetic surgery.

What was the initial feeling that made you begin to consider cosmetic surgery and look through this book? What part of you bothers you? Try standing in front of a full-length mirror or using a magnifying mirror with a bright light to look at yourself carefully, and think about how you'd really feel if you could improve any part of your physical self that leaves you spiritually and emotionally dissatisfied. Do you have isolated pockets of flab that just won't go away, no matter how hard you diet and exercise? You might want to consider one of the new varieties of liposuction. Are you bothered by creased horizontal lines and droop on the forehead that make you look tired, sad, or worried? We now have mini-browlifts that can improve those lines and lift that brow away. Do you have harsh vertical lines between the eyebrows that make you look angry? There are new methods of treatment that work like magic—Botox, SoftForm, and fat-transfer.

We've got traditional procedures like rhinoplasty for people

unhappy with their noses; breast enlargement, lift, and reduction for those unhappy with the look of their breasts; and classic facelifts to fix the tired, droopy look. But now we've also got
laser skin resurfacing if you have serious, deep wrinkles, scars,
and discolorations; laser eyelid lifts for hooded or raccoon-
saucer eyes; and microsuction to fix a jowly turkey neck.

If you've always thought that cosmetic surgery meant a wind-
blown, "deer caught in the headlights" look, guess again. Most
of my patients swear that no one knows they've had anything
done unless they've been told. The chart below and the chapters
that follow will detail exactly what the latest revolution in cosmetic surgery can do for you.

PERMANENT FLAB (see chapter 10)

Traditional liposuction	Liposculption
reduces large bulges only	reduces large bulges and allows delicate sculpting of muscle groups for "six-pack" athletic look
can only be done on people with tight skin to begin with	can be done on people with loose skin and can actually tighten loose skin
can only work on limited areas	can sculpt the whole torso
kills fat that is removed	fat removed is alive and can be reinjected to improve wrinkles, enhance cheeks, chins, and even lift the buttocks
more incisions	fewer incisions

WRINKLES, SCARS, AND DISCOLORATIONS
(see chapter 7)

Deep peel/dermabrasion	Carbon dioxide laser
uses chemicals or mechanical devices with often unpredictable results	uses space age science to improve imperfections in the skin
doctor has less control of the depth of injury	doctor has complete control over depth
very painful, recovery four to six weeks	almost never painful, recovery two to four weeks
can permanently lose facial pigment leading to an alabaster look	pigment loss very rare; leaves skin soft, velvety with a healthy glow
cost: $5,000 to $7,000 (more visits required)	the same cost, but fewer visits

THINNING HAIR AND BALD SPOTS
(see chapter 5)

Traditional plugs	"Sushi" hair transplant
not possible for most women or profoundly bald men	possible for both, as one to three hairs are transplanted individually
two-week recovery	two- to six-day recovery
artificial picket-fence look	totally natural looking
cost: up to $25,000 for the severely bald	cost: $8,000 to $12,000

JOWLY, DROOPY LOOK (see chapter 9)

Traditional upper facelift	Alternative facelift
all or nothing procedure	breaks down facial surgery into smaller procedures catering to individual needs
long painful recovery (three to six weeks)	short, often painless recovery (four to seven days)
large bandages; often visible scars	no bandages; smaller, less visible scars
can yield a wind-tunnel, pulled look	very natural result
cost: $12,000 to $20,000	cost: $4,500 to $7,000

TIRED, HOUND-DOG EYES (see chapter 8)

Scalpel eyelid lift	Carbon dioxide eyelid lift
Scalpel means more bruising, bleeding	virtually no bleeding and bruising
ten- to fourteen-day recovery	four- to seven-day recovery
usually leaves a visible scar that can be permanent	lower eyelids can be done without any incision or scar on the skin
often leaves eyes unnaturally round	leaves eyes naturally shaped
cost: approximately $3,000	cost: approximately $2,500

TURKEY NECK (see chapter 4)

Traditional lower facelift	Microsuction
often leaves a pulled, wind-tunnel look	yields a completely natural look

involves long incisions and scars	no cutting, pulling, or sewing
at least seven to fourteen days hiding at home	can go back to work in one or two days
requires major anesthesia	local anesthesia only
cost: about $10,000 or more	one-third the cost

If you're reading this book because you're thinking of taking the first steps toward surgery and feeling nervous and unsure, you're not alone. Answering your questions and discussing your fears is what a consultation with a cosmetic surgeon is for, and you'll learn exactly what that process entails in chapter 3, "How to Choose a Doctor." In the chapters that follow, you'll also learn about many of my patients' experiences with the new cosmetic surgery techniques, and will look at their before-and-after photographs to see for yourself what the results can be. For now, though, you should consider what one woman, Bev Oberg, had to say:

> Once you break through that "not sure" level, once you meet the doctors and understand the techniques, and that the downtime is really very small and the cost is reasonable, all you can think is: "What took me so long?"
>
> I had sun damage around the eyes from living in Arizona and San Diego and just wanted to lightly erase what fifty-one years had put on my face, but I didn't want anyone to say, "Oh look at her, she must've had this and this done." When I saw what laser surgery did for my friend Joyce, I knew I had to have it too.
>
> I went in on a Thursday and was back at work on Monday, and I may have looked a little odd, but it was amazing to people that it could be done so easily. It's just enhancing what you had and getting it back and I think for those of us in our fifties, that's really important. We are still active and still busy and still have careers, and if we're out in the workforce, it gives us so much more confidence. It not only lifts your face—it lifts your spirits.

Part One

THE NEW AESTHETIC SURGERY

✳

Chapter 1

WHEN VANITY IS NOT A SIN

THE HISTORY AND PSYCHOLOGY OF AESTHETIC SURGERY

You know the TV ads that say, "I'm not only the president of Hair Club for Men; I'm also a client"? Well, my becoming a dermatologist in the first place was just like that—a case of "physician, heal thyself." Back as far as anyone can remember, my family has had a history of extreme eczema (dry skin), which may sound funny as a family curse until you realize that, in cases where more than half your body's skin is involved, life can become a torment. Besides scabies, eczema is the only rash with an itch so strong it can wake you up out of a sound sleep, and it's not uncommon for sufferers to scratch themselves bloody.

My mother was so afflicted with eczema that she almost died from it, and I was born with the same condition. One of my earliest childhood memories is of large patches of my skin being itchy, red, and scaly. My mom had a whole medicine chest full of old-fashioned, smelly, and greasy creams she would put on my dry skin to try to soothe it. I was so embarrassed by the condition that I'd wear long-sleeved shirts to school—in New York City, in July!

At Yale med school, by pure coincidence, my faculty advisor was Marty Carter, a Ph.D. in biochemistry and a professor of dermatology. With the terrible stress of med school my skin went into overdrive, and I was a regular at the Yale Derm clinic. I ended up becoming a case history for the staff, the chairman, and even Marty himself, each trying the latest techniques on my world-class eczema. They were all the greatest people you could ever hope to meet, and I was so taken with everyone there that I fell in love with dermatology and haven't looked back since. Besides, if you've got a hereditary case of chronic skin trouble like mine, the only way you can afford a dermatologist for you and your family is to *be* one.

So I'm not only a dermatologist and a cosmetic surgeon; I'm also a consumer of both dermatology and cosmetic surgery. My parents were in their forties when I was born, which was very unusual at that time, and I remember growing up and thinking that my mom and dad were older looking than the other parents in the neighborhood. In my earliest memories of my mother and father, they were already middle-aged, and when I started to look as my parents had looked when I was young, I started having twinges, the twinges you get when you look in the mirror and feel so much younger than you look. This is something that almost everyone coming in for a surgery consultation says to me—that they look so old on the outside but *feel* so young on the inside.

My son Alan Jr. was born when I was forty-three. We ride bicycles, roller blade, play tennis, and golf together, and being a stereotypic Californian, I am a very serious exercise guy, getting an all-out aerobic workout three times a week for the past fifteen years. I am fifty-three years old now, one of the oldest of the boomers, and a few years ago, my son and I attended a parent-teacher conference at his school—a conference where the teachers and other parents there all chimed in on how lucky little Alan was that his grandfather had come to visit. Is it any wonder that, right afterward, I got an alternative mini-facelift and a fat transfer? Now, whenever I see a friend, patient, or colleague I haven't seen in a while, there's always the same comment: "You've never looked better!" But not only have I never looked better, more importantly, I've never *felt* better.

When you read the stories later in this book of my patients, who have generously shared with you why they had cosmetic surgery and what effect it has had on their lives, I think you will know something I have always known. Fifty years ago, cosmetic surgery was primarily for the rich and famous. Now, more than a million Americans a year are doing it, and these are people just like you and me. More than ever before, cosmetic surgery has become a practical and necessary adjunct to life, but far more importantly, cosmetic surgery resonates from some of the deepest, most important and even spiritual parts of us. It gets to the heart of how we feel about ourselves.

All cosmetic surgery begins when people identify a problem in their appearance that they wish to correct, changing the outside to bring it into harmony with the inside. An improved appearance—a more attractive and likeable you—will almost always lead to such changes as greater confidence and a better overall mood and feeling. When people feel their best, they're always more able to do their best and have far more to give to others.

One of my patients, Anna Ramirez, told me that she was in a relationship for fifteen years, then

the guy suddenly got married to somebody else, so I was at a certain point in my life where I didn't exactly feel good about myself. It got to the point where I didn't even want to look at myself in the mirror, I looked so sad all the time, like a seventy-year-old woman. It wasn't like after the surgery I was expecting to see a movie star—I just wanted to see myself again.

I finally went and did it: laser wrinkle removal, neck microsuction, minilift. I could've gone back to work the third day, but instead I took two weeks' vacation and then told everyone when

I came back that it was just being away from the office that made me look so good. The changes were so completely natural that nobody knew I had had any kind of surgery or facelift at all; they couldn't even guess. They kept saying how rested and great I looked and I loved hearing it. It definitely changed everything I think about myself. It really was an all-new me.

You know how everyone's looking for the fountain of youth? I think Dr. Gaynor's found it.

When I opened my practice in 1980 with another just-starting dermatologist, I was removing skin cancers and life-threatening moles, while my partner was using the collagen-injection treatment to improve facial wrinkles that he'd learned during his dermatology training at Stanford. At one point he taught me how to perform the technique, and I couldn't believe the difference it made in my patients. Of course people were grateful when harmful growths and moles were removed, but those who had wrinkles temporarily improved with collagen injections were sincerely happy, with an extra bounce in their step. Seeing this simple procedure make such a change in my patients' and my (yes, I had collagen shots back then, too) outlook on life made me reconsider my own work and launched me into the extra training and schooling I needed to become a cosmetic surgeon.

Beauty may be only "skin deep," but that thin layer of skin is awfully important in almost all our interactions as human beings. Think of children's fairy tales, where the witch is always wicked, old, and ugly while the prince and princess are always good, young, and beautiful. People generally think that those with good looks have better, more glamorous lives, and anyone who's ever socialized with a beautiful woman (who gets into clubs without waiting in line, or even paying, and can frequently talk her way out of a traffic ticket) can see this prejudice in action. More than we may want to admit, looks matter.

The importance of beauty is felt as early as infancy and

preschool. A 1980 University of Michigan study involved four-
to six-month-old babies who, while sitting on their mothers'
laps, were shown slide projections of attractive and less attractive faces. The infants spent more time looking at the attractive
faces and smiled more often at these faces.

Two other Michigan studies used photographs of attractive
and less attractive children and adults and asked preschool children to indicate which person was most likely to be nicer and
which person they would most like to play with. Consistently,
young children labeled attractive individuals as nicer than those
who were deemed less attractive (though they showed no difference in their play choices).

Recent investigation suggests that a baby's physical appearance has profound implications on how he or she is treated. For
example, nurses in a ward of premature babies were asked to rate
infants' intellectual capacities. Almost every time, the more attractive children were felt to be of higher intelligence than the
less attractive infants. Another study asked college students to
judge a child's personal character after the child had seriously
misbehaved. Physically attractive children were thought to be
tired, cranky, hungry, or just having an off day, while unattractive children were judged as having deep-seated personality dis-
orders. Research also shows that attractive children are punished
less often and are kissed, cuddled, and smiled at more often than
unattractive ones.

Is it any wonder that with all of these psychological and social pressures, more and more Americans are seeking cosmetic
surgery? In 1965, researchers at Johns Hopkins Hospital reported that 85 percent of facelift patients had an improved sense
of well being, a greater sense of social ease, and were less self-
critical of themselves and others after surgery. Of the patients
who were clearly depressed, most showed improvement postoperatively. Most striking was that a quarter of the patients reported salary raises, awards, and new or better jobs, which they
attributed to their enhanced appearance. About half described

positive changes in their personal lives that included the formation of new or better relationships or the termination of old unsatisfactory relationships.

Ellen Berscheid, in *Psychological Aspects of Facial Form,* summed
it all up:

> I suspect that the growth in importance of physical attractiveness
> in today's society is partly due to our increased geographic mo-
> bility, as well as the concentration of our population in large ur-
> ban areas. Because of these factors, people are now meeting more
> people in casual encounters than ever before. For example, it is
> estimated that the average twenty-year-old entering the job mar-
> ket will change jobs at least seven times during their working
> years. The divorce rate has risen over 700 percent since the turn
> of the century. In a society in which one cannot even count on
> having the same set of parents in our childhood for any length of
> time; the same marriage partner for any length of time; when one
> may be thrown in to the dating and mating market at age thirty,
> forty, fifty, sixty; when it becomes increasingly unlikely that one
> will have the same workmates, colleagues, or neighbors for any
> length of time—in sum, in a society in which social fragmenta-
> tion has proceeded to an unprecedented point, people are con-
> stantly assessed very quickly by others simply on the basis of
> their appearance rather than upon their record of actual behavior
> and other characteristics. Is it any wonder, then, that to help
> them cope, people look to the new keepers of the fountain of
> beauty and youth—the cosmetic surgeons, the dentists, the nu-
> tritionists, the cosmeticians, the physical therapists, and so on?

Over the past twenty years I've done thousands of consults,
and a huge percentage of those patients tell me they actually
feel guilty wanting to change their looks. You, the man or
woman considering cosmetic surgery, are more likely than not
to be uncomfortable that you want to look your best; you think
it's embarrassing to be so vain that you're coming to a surgeon
for help.

What you must remember is that the desire to be more beautiful, to look one's best, is as ancient as the human race. Since the beginning of recorded time, men and women have searched for the fountain of youth, for ways to reverse the inevitable effects of aging. They've applied various substances to their faces and bodies in an effort to ensure that their skin stay vigorous, elastic, lustrous, and youthful. The legendary seductress Cleopatra used milk in her baths and peeled her skin with lactic acid, which is very similar to the glycolic acid that is so popular today. The women of the African Bantu forest still apply mud to their faces (as their ancestors have done for eons), and the ancient nomads, who settled along the Nile between 10,000 and 5,000 B.C., used cosmetics to protect their skin from the sun.

Ancient peoples actively imported and exported eye paint, perfumes, and ointments as a significant means of commerce. At the dawn of ancient Egypt, black antimony powder was used to shape and color the eyebrows, lead sulfide was used to outline and accentuate the eyes, while green malachite was applied to the eyelid as shadow. In fact, most of the cosmetics we use today women used centuries ago, tinting their fingernails and toenails, applying rouge to their lips and cheeks, and dyeing or bleaching their hair. When Egyptian Queen Nefertiti's tomb was unearthed, archaeologists found a bronze mirror, gold cosmetic cases, hairpins, tweezers, rouge pots, kohl (used for mascara), and ointments that had retained their scent.

Ancient Egyptians lived in a fertile desert, and a key part of their concept of beauty centered on smooth, beautiful skin. The Ebers papyrus, dated at 2,000 B.C., describes a host of various medical techniques, including a primitive dermabrasion (the smoothing of wrinkles or scars): "To make skin smooth take water from the gebu plant, meal of alabaster, and fresh Abt grain. Mix in honey and make into a pap [like baby food]. Then mix in human milk and anoint the face therewith." The Smith papyrus, of around 4,000 B.C., describes methods of dealing with wounds and scars, with particular attention given to cosmetic results. Large wounds were stitched, while smaller ones were bound together with strips of adhesive plaster. This papyrus also alludes to the use of naturally occurring anesthetics so that surgeons could perform more intricate, painful surgeries at minimal discomfort to the patient. A solution derived from Indian hemp was an incredibly effective pain reliever and was in use more than four thousand years ago!

Cosmetic surgery is one of the oldest forms of medicine, with a history measured in thousands of years. The earliest cosmetic surgery, in fact, served to alter the body in ways we certainly don't find beautiful today. The Tartars of western Russia admired flat broad noses and so bandaged any child's nose that had the bolder "Roman" profile that is more suited to contemporary ideals of beauty. A similar attitude was found in the Maya of Central America, who thought crossed eyes and flat noses were beautiful and so tied up a developing child's nose with a board while dangling a stone from a string in front of the child's eyes. Another example is the ancient Chinese practice of binding girls' feet. According to the Chinese, a girl with small, dainty feet was the ideal of beauty. Further, bound feet demonstrated the wealth of a family because a girl with bound feet couldn't walk and needed to be carried long distances.

In the past, physical alteration as a punishment for crime was not uncommon: noses, ears, and hands were cut off. In the India of 1,500 B.C., for example, a husband or father, without direct proof, had the right to cut off a woman's nose if she was thought to be unchaste or unfaithful. As one can well imagine, many women were unjustly punished, and in the rare case when a man would later admit his mistake, the nose would be repaired—the first reconstructive surgery (or "nose jobs") in recorded history. The Hindus were not alone; ancient Egyptians practiced disfigurement as well, with skilled surgeons who could amputate without endangering the accused's life. These same surgeons were sometimes called upon to repair people who had been unjustly punished.

During the Middle Ages, however, physical beauty was not appreciated, especially in women. It was believed that beauty would lure otherwise God-fearing men into the arms of the devil, and performing cosmetic surgery could actually be punishable by death. This attitude, in various forms and degrees, would last for the next four hundred years, until the sixteenth century brought a widespread epidemic of syphilis to Europe. One effect of untreated syphilis is a drastic deformation of the nose, which caused great shame among those who had the unfortunate luck of contracting the disease. It was so common, in fact, that the nose became a sign of morality, with those affected immediately labeled as immoral individuals who deserved to walk around for life with a disfigured appearance for their sinful ways. Understandably, this stigma rekindled interest in cosmetic surgery, and it was under these conditions, in 1597, that the Italian doctor Gaspare Tagliacozzi (often called the father of cosmetic surgery) wrote a guide that systematically outlined the surgical grafting of the nose and ears. His fame became so great that the city of Bologna built a statue of Dr. Tagliacozzi holding a nose in his hand.

It must be remembered that surgeries during this time were very primitive. There was little understanding of how infection occurred, and anesthetics weren't readily available (the knowledge regarding use of herbal medicines and drugs to dull pain had been lost through the centuries). Anyone who endured surgery had to be a very brave soul indeed, one who was not only ready to endure tremendous pain, but also ready for (more often than not) terrible results. Tagliacozzi was also one of the first to allude to the psychological effects on patients of having such surgeries: "We restore, repair, and make whole those parts of the face which Nature has given but which Fortune has taken away, not so much that they may delight the eye but that they may buoy up the spirit and help the mind of the afflicted." These words, four hundred years old, remain true of my own work today.

In the last one hundred years, surgery as a whole has under-gone a dramatic evolution. Sophisticated pain management is now taken for granted, recovery periods for even the most ex-tensive techniques can be counted in days, and bad outcomes are rare when the work is done with good skill and technique. What is almost equally remarkable, however, is that the attitude toward cosmetic surgery, both with doctors themselves and with the general public, has taken a full 180-degree turn. What has happened in modern society, for the first time since practically the ancient Egyptians, to make cosmetic surgery not only ac-cepted but sought after by millions of men and women each year? It was nothing less than war.

The First World War was unlike any previously fought, in that all the power of modern scientific advances was used to create bullets, bombs, tanks, and poisonous gasses that had unprece-dented ability to kill, disfigure, and maim. With machine guns pumping thousands of bullets per minute and bombs that were larger and more dangerous than ever before, the hundreds of thousands of men who fought in the trenches and who were not killed outright were seriously disfigured, and lice and bacteria-infested mud caused soldiers to get terrible infections in their wounds that led to further deformity—all in the preantibiotic era.

The injuries endured by these brave men were more extensive than had ever been seen before. Those who lived (and the num-ber was impressive because general surgery was, by necessity, advancing quickly) were often maimed beyond recognition. Many could never hope to regain a normal place in society. His-torically, cosmetically minded general surgeons were interested mainly in rebuilding the lost or deformed body part. However, with wounds as atrocious as those suffered by these soldiers, consideration began to be given to aesthetic results. While out-comes weren't nearly as good as they are today, the work of these surgeons showed that even a person whose face had once been terribly injured could be partly or completely restored so that they could resume a normal life. This surgery was performed by general surgeons. Plastic surgery, per se, did not exist until the late 1940s, when the demand for aesthetic results increased and cosmetically minded surgeons began to focus exclusively on this type of surgery.

The next great impetus to advance aesthetic surgery came from the changing nature of the workplace, when thousands of workers were injured and disfigured by the new machines of the Industrial Revolution. These accidents could produce damage as extensive as those seen in war, and early twentieth-century cosmetic surgeons used the skills they had perfected in the trenches for these victims of technology. But as little as fifty years ago, society drew a strong distinction between surgery undertaken to fix injured people and surgery to reverse aging or improve appearance, such as "fixing" an unattractive nose. It was more acceptable in the time of Cleopatra to improve appearance just for the pleasure and joy of looking your best than it was in 1920.

The modern acceptance of cosmetic surgery as a way to improve the appearance of anyone who wanted it finally occurred during the Roaring Twenties. Unfortunately, many of the procedures performed by doctors, lay people, and out-and-out quacks at this time were still dangerous, with many nonmedically trained charlatans performing untested, outlandish methods.

One example was the use of paraffin (wax) injections, which became the rage for treating facial wrinkles. This treatment involved the injection of paraffin into the stretched folds of wrinkled skin, especially of wrinkles around the mouth. After some time, the wax would set and produce adequate results, at least in the short term. Long term, however, the paraffin would move, causing deformities, while the wrinkles that were initially treated would reappear and, all too commonly, the injection site would become so inflamed and tender that even the slightest touch could cause agony. If the patient wasn't immediately treated, infection would occur, sometimes resulting in vast amounts of skin tissue being shed, leading to huge facial deformities. These terrible results were so common during the twenties that they became known as the "paraffin menace."

Despite quack procedures like the paraffin technique, those who believed in cosmetic surgery persisted in their endeavors throughout the twentieth century. Vast bodies of knowledge began to be assembled, shared, and written down by reputable doctors. This was the first step toward the making of a profession. Experiments were carried out in large numbers and doctors performed as many purely aesthetic operations as they could.

World War II brought about a complete revolution in attitude toward cosmetic surgery. For the first time, no patient was discharged until every cosmetic repair had been made as fully as possible. Front-line surgeons were taught ways to sew wounds to leave as small a scar as possible. New drugs that minimized infection, namely penicillin and sulfa, became readily available, allowing wounds to heal more reliably and predictably. Some cosmetic surgeons were deliberately altering people's faces so that they might work more closely with the resistance movements as spies behind enemy lines.

In the 1990s, the field of cosmetic surgery is treated just like any other medical specialty. The growth of surgical technique over the past fifty years, and the current understanding that anyone who wants to change their looks should be allowed to do so without shame or embarrassment, is nothing more than our modern version of the timeless desire to look as attractive as possible. After all my years of experience in the field, I am certain that the urge to look as good as you can has been hardwired into human consciousness since the beginning of time. Just think, with all our current techniques, what a great beauty Cleopatra could be today.

[Assistance in writing and research from Beth Gaynor]

Chapter 2

DON'T JUST STAND THERE—DO IT YOURSELF!

METHODS YOU CAN USE TO KEEP YOUR SKIN HEALTHY

Of all the television shows I've appeared on over the years, my favorites by far are the many variations on the theme of doctors' home remedies. In these segments, I show the audience various products readily available at discount drugstores and supermarkets that can effectively treat common skin problems. Today there are creams and lotions, for example, that treat athlete's foot and even severely dry skin, and you can now buy them for the first time without a prescription. Many are low priced, and others will save you a visit to the dermatologist, so these kinds of tips may not be the best promotion for my business, but they are great for your pocketbook.

Several years ago I was doing this type of show with a well-known bodybuilder and workout personality. I'd brought to the studio over-the-counter products that could treat such maladies as eczema (dry skin), psoriasis, athlete's foot, and even head lice, and all of them were inexpensive, nonprescription, and practical. Usually, before a show like this, I get a few minutes of the host's time to brief him or her about the topic so as to prevent a disaster on camera. Well, every time I tried to speak to this particular host, we were interrupted as he signed receipts for the shipping of workout suits he was selling by the tens of thousands (which made me wonder for just a moment if I'd chosen the wrong career).

The show started, I was going through disease after disease on camera, finally getting to the remedies for psoriasis (a generally harmless skin problem where red scale builds up, usually on the knees and elbows), and before I could open my mouth, the host said, "Dr. Gaynor, I see next you'll be telling us all about home remedies to treat cirrhosis (liver disease)." It was funny, but I really squirmed on camera getting out of that goof.

Unfortunately, there aren't any doctors' home remedies for cirrhosis just yet, but there are plenty for psoriasis and other skin troubles. There are also plenty of inexpensive, but very effective, products you can get and techniques you can follow to keep your skin as young and healthy as it can be. Follow these methods, and maybe you can even put off needing to see someone like me for a while.

Let's start with the crucial question: What is human skin? It's the body's biggest (and I think the most beautiful) organ; it protects you, cushions you, insulates you, and provides you with the elements of sensory information. As a dermatologist, I believe it is the most wonderful body part.

Skin has three layers. The top, the epidermis, is the part you see and feel, with a surface made up entirely of dead cells. As you age, the natural sloughing off of these dead cells slows, making skin look tired. Dermabrasion, chemical peel, and laser skin resurfacing greatly improve the look of skin by removing the old layers, allowing the new skin to rebuild itself with fresh, new cells.

The dermis, just underneath, is the home of sweat glands, hair follicles, collagen, and elastin fibers (which are like rubber bands) that give the skin its tightness, toughness, firmness, and elastic strength. With age, gravity will slowly loosen the elastin and collagen fibers, leading to the characteristic droop and slackness we see in the skin of older people. The only way to avoid these changes is to spend your life on a planet or space station with zero gravity. In spite of what you may have heard or read, no cream containing collagen or elastin is ever going to soak through the skin to make it young and tight again.

The third layer of the skin, the subcutis, is made up of the fat that feeds and supports the top two layers. The subcutis also cushions and insulates you from the outside world. We may not like having too much body fat, but not having any at all would never work and would be very unattractive. So much of the beauty, roundness, and softness that makes human bodies so lovely to behold comes from the underlying fat. As we age we naturally lose some of this fat, leading to, for example, the mummified look of old hands and thin necks.

The skin of a baby generally is very soft, velvety, all one color, and certainly free of wrinkles, blemishes, and liver spots. How wonderful it would be if our skin stayed this way our whole lives. By the time we reach puberty, most of us have already significantly damaged our skin from unprotected sun exposure, and if that weren't bad enough, at puberty oil (sebaceous) glands start up, our pores widen, and most of us develop acne. These changes are caused by the turning on of the male and female hormones responsible for so many of the exciting differences between men and women. As we age and progress through life, the skin continues to age with us. It dries and itches and its color becomes irregular (with freckling, age spots, and moles), and the blood vessels dilate. Some of these changes are unavoidable, but others will respond to intervention if you begin early enough.

The Sun

Like the calories we eat, every bit of unprotected sun exposure we get is remembered and counted by the skin. Almost all parents use those adorable sunbonnets with large visors on newborn babies, but after six months or a year, most of us skip the bonnets and just put our kids on the beach and around swimming pools with little or no protection. By the time we are in our thirties and forties and see the sun blotches, liver spots, and wrinkles from the sun on our faces, we finally wake up and start using sun lotions and large-brimmed hats, and we even find the shade a much nicer place to sit. By that age, however—though it's never too late to protect our skin—a great deal of damage has already been done.

The great majority of sun damage, in fact, happens in the first twenty years of life. How many of you who are now over twenty-one even have the time to bake in the sun? When my family moved from New York City to sunny Fort Lauderdale, I'd always be the very first person to arrive at the pool every morning and, like a plant, I'd turn my chair to face the damaging rays all day long.

The wrinkles, liver spots, and even skin cancers caused by the sun usually don't show up for twenty or thirty years. The time to deal with this problem, however, is when our children are born. We should always and without exception protect their skin by using sunscreen lotions and hats and by keeping them in the shade. Doing this from birth is the greatest thing you can do to profoundly slow the visible signs of aging and prevent skin cancers, especially on the face. People spend billions of dollars a year on cosmetic surgery and creams to reverse wrinkles and liver spots, much of which would be unnecessary if they'd protected themselves from the sun earlier in life.

I know what you're thinking (doctors always like to think they can read their patients' minds)—that you shouldn't take beach vacations, go out for bike rides, play tennis or golf, or enjoy the warmth of the sun on an early spring day after a hard winter. Nothing could be further from the truth, but there are certain facts about the sun and your skin that are worth remembering, starting with the most important: skin color. Nature had it right—people living close to the equator evolved darker skin over hundreds of thousands of years as a natural sun protection. I once spent six months living in London and remember only a handful of clear, warm, sunny days. No wonder people whose ancestors came from there evolved very light skin to catch the little bit of sun available and maximize the body's production of vitamin D (which is made in the skin). Transplant those people to sunny California, where I live now, and their light skin, which provides almost no natural sun protection, rapidly ages to look like those California raisins that used to dance across our television screens. If your skin and hair are light and your eyes are blue, the sun will wreck your skin and make you look prematurely old far faster than if you're Mediterranean, Asian, or African-American. So all I have to say about this issue goes double for the famed California blonds.

Second, the time of day at which you are exposed to the sun is crucial. When the sun is low on the horizon in the early morning or late afternoon, its ability to harm the skin is dramatically less than when it is directly overhead from eleven to three. In fact, it is on those workdays when we go walking in the sun at lunchtime and on those weekends when we play outdoors all day and never think to use sunscreens or hats that the vast amount of yearly sun damage occurs. This damage easily can be greater than that which occurs on a sunny vacation day when we remember to cover up.

Third, sitting next to a swimming pool, swimming in the ocean, or skiing at high altitudes greatly magnifies the sun's harmful effects, both because of reflection and from a thinner atmosphere; for every thousand feet of elevation, there's roughly a 4 percent increase in sun damage. This means that at five thousand feet of elevation, the effects of the sun will be 20 percent greater than at sea level. Some prescription medications, such as certain antibiotics, birth control pills, high blood pressure medication and even some acne pills, can intensify sun damage. You should always ask your doctor if your prescription can have this effect.

Knowing all this, is it my professional opinion that you should never go outside when the sun is out and live like some kind of hermit? Of course not. You can have your cake and eat it, too, if you practice some very simple techniques. The first, and most important, is the religious use of sunscreens. Start your babies on them; teach them to apply them on their own as soon as they can; and set a good example by using them yourselves.

The SPF, or sun protection factor—numbers on sun lotion bottles—means a lot: the higher the number, the greater the protection. Many manufacturers claim that their products are "retentive," meaning they'll stick to the skin even in the water or when you sweat. Don't count on it. I tell my patients that they should reapply sun lotions every time they go in the water, after every set of tennis, and after every few ski runs down the mountain. I even think it's very important to put on a little protection if you know you'll be outside for any extended period of time in the wintertime. A good bottle of SPF 29 sun lotion (which will afford plenty of protection to even the fairest skins) should cost under ten dollars at supermarkets and discount drug stores. All sun lotions with an SPF of 29 are equal; keep it simple and cheap when you buy them, and you can easily skip shopping in the high-end boutiques. An average-sized bottle of sun lotion should only last a few weekends if you lead an outdoor life. If it lasts all summer, you're not applying it often enough and you need to put it on more frequently. And remember that sunscreen also loses its potency if it sits on the shelf for too long. It can become ineffective and "go bad" within one or two years.

Check the ingredients on sun lotion bottles carefully. Several decades ago, products like zinc oxide were used for sun protection, but they made you look like you'd spilled paint on your face. Then came PABA, which was cosmetically acceptable but highly allergenic. Dermatologists like me had a brisk summertime business treating the rashes PABA gave many users. Still, it was a great advance, because it was invisible. Currently, you should look for sun lotions that have several ingredients (such as benzophenones, cinnamates, and titanium dioxide), each of which protects you from a particular spectrum of the harmful rays of the sun. Speak to your dermatologist or the pharmacist at your local discount drug store for advice on which product is best for you.

You can be completely protected from the sun's harmful rays, but at a price. How many of us are willing to brag about going on a sunny vacation in the winter to our friends and coworkers, and then come back as pale and pasty as when we left? The answer is to use the newly available and perfectly natural tanning lotions that you leave on overnight and wake looking like you had the vacation of your dreams, even if it rained so hard during your trip that you never saw a speck of sun.

Tanning products come in several forms, but all of them work the same way, safely and temporarily adding color with makeup dyes. There are bronzing gels, which directly apply pigment to the skin and work well as long as you stand perfectly still, don't sweat, and live in a climate with no heat or humidity. The minute you do anything, many of these products streak, run, and make your skin look like the pattern seen in burl wood. Bronzing powders work a bit better than the gels, but the best are tanning accelerators that actually produce a credible-looking tan. The beauty is that these cause absolutely no damage to the skin. Remember, apply these evenly or you will see hand and finger marks until the color fades several days later.

The funny thing about all this is that, before the 1900s, the ultimate sign of negative social status you could have was to sport a tan. Rich people wouldn't be caught dead with a tan because they could afford to sit inside and watch the poor people working in the fields, exposed to the sun as they worked. It was after the Industrial Revolution, when poor people began working in factories, that this whole system turned topsy-turvy. Poor people became as sallow as rich people, creating a genuine social dilemma.

Along came Coco Chanel, the great French couturier. In 1914 she went to the French Riviera, came back with a tan, pronounced that tan was in, and this is when the "tan is healthy, and healthy is cool" concept began. A tan now proved that one had the time and wealth to sit in the sun, and those of us with weather-beaten, sun-damaged, wrinkled skin (and even skin cancer) are living with the consequences.

There is only one technique to slow the aging of the face, and now you know what it is—avoiding the rays of the sun. The only other factors that determine the speed of aging are smoking and genetics. Look at your parents' photos; if they aged gracefully, you will as well, and only the sun can really make it otherwise.

Many of my patients want to know if tanning parlors are safe, and I always want to respond, "Safer than what?" If you're asking whether tanning parlors are safer than going into direct sunlight, then yes, they probably are. The ultraviolet rays from the sun are the ones that make the skin age and cause cancer, while the wonderful infrared rays (that keep us warm) and visible rays (that let us read important books like this one) are thought to be harmless. The ultraviolet rays come in several forms: B rays cause sunburns and are the most damaging to the skin, while A rays make your skin tan. Though the As harm the skin as well, they're weaker and harm it more slowly.

I suppose there's a strange logic that tanning parlors try to use to convince people of their relative safety. In their advertising, they often say that because their lightbulbs only put out the tanning A rays, they are safer than sunbathing. In the most limited sense, this is correct. My view is that tanning parlors give people wrinkles and skin cancer more slowly than direct sunlight, but they surely do terrible damage over time.

There is just no such thing as a safe tan; in fact, tanning is the skin's way of protecting itself against a toxic overexposure of light. Getting and maintaining a tan through machines is dangerous and does terrible lifetime damage to your skin. Though not bossy by nature, in good conscience, I must advise you never to go to tanning parlors. I hope you will listen.

Moisturizers

Moisturizers, per se, will not remove wrinkles and liver spots permanently, but they can have the wonderful temporary effect of making the skin smooth and soft. Moisturizers do this by sealing in the skin's own moisture, very much like paint protecting a wall. These products do improve the texture and feel of the skin. They can even help smooth very fine wrinkles for a short time. But a plain nonprescription product cannot penetrate deeply enough, by law, to do more than this. Over the years, many catch-all ingredients have been added to moisturizers to increase sales and prices. Ingredients such as collagen, elastin, placenta, aloe vera, and others are being prominently mentioned as key formulations in the products sold by virtually all the large cosmetic companies. As advertised in full page ads in *Vogue, Allure,* and other magazines, these products sport names and promotional copy that imply or even state that they can lift, rejuvenate, or protect the skin, or even improve the skin's strength (I'm not even sure what that means). The question I am often asked is whether these ingredients do anything beyond what a well-made, inexpensive product like Vaseline Intensive Care does, and the answer is an unequivocal no.

Over the years I have watched in amazement as the utterly false and deceptive claims made by such products have escalated faster than the national debt. Anyone buying these cosmetics would have to be convinced by the packaging that the ingredients that make them so expensive will do something wonderful. The truth is that there is no medical, scientific, or common sense evidence to prove that these products do anything more for your skin than can be accomplished with the olive oil from your kitchen cabinet. What these products lift, rejuvenate, and protect are the corporate profits of the companies that manufacture them.

Later in this chapter I will be discussing exciting new ingredients such as antioxidants (vitamin C), glycolic acid, betahydroxy acids, and others that hold some promise of improving the appearance of the skin. Even though dermatologists are just beginning to evaluate whether these chemicals do, in fact, have a small but noticeable effect on liver spots and fine wrinkles, the last way in the world I'd use them would be through products in full-page national women's magazine advertisements. If vitamin C in moisturizer turns out to improve the skin (not remotely proven for now, by the way), I would personally wait until it was available in a generic, inexpensive moisturizer such as those found in discount drugstores or supermarkets.

Save your money and keep it simple and inexpensive when buying moisturizers. When any ad seeks to imply a direct medical effect, yet the product still does not need any government regulation, you should be suspicious. The next time one of these "revolutionary" products is announced, read the ads very carefully and notice how the language hedges. If any of these products, now marketed as "cosmeceuticals," were to actually make medical claims, they'd have to be approved by the FDA. One of the dermatologists who helped develop a new vitamin C–based cream said it best: "When it comes right down to it, a lot of these things are just hope in a jar."

When choosing these products, think about what you are trying to accomplish. If your skin is naturally dry, the use of a moisturizer to seal in and hold on to the little bit of moisture your skin can make is a great idea. If your skin is oily to begin with, applying a moisturizer can make it downright greasy, and then you will have to go out and spend money on an astringent to remove the oil. Many cosmetic routines take advantage of this dog-chasing-its-tail approach to skin care, selling a moisturizer to someone who doesn't need it, and then selling a bunch of other products to remove the grease and even to treat the acne and plugged pores caused by the moisturizer that was never needed in the first place.

One of the most-believed consumer myths is that people with dry skin are more likely to prematurely wrinkle than people with oily skin, but this is just not true. What happens is that almost all of us notice our skin getting drier as we age, about the same time we would have noticed wrinkles anyway. The dry skin doesn't cause the wrinkles; it's just another sign of aging. Lifetime use of moisturizers will not slow or delay wrinkles, which actually come from sun exposure, smoking, facial expression, and, most significantly, genes.

My skin has always been drier than a potato chip, and so I use moisturizers on my body especially after bathing, but I've never bought a moisturizer that cost more than $10 for a big bottle, and neither should you. In fact, the most popular "moisturizer" during the Great Depression of the 1930s is said to have been Crisco shortening. On a TV appearance I took a small can of Crisco and wrapped it in brown paper, obscuring the label. I then applied a small bit of the Crisco to the back of the hand of the very elegant host. I asked her if it felt greasy, and she said no. I asked her to smell it—Crisco is unscented—and she said it smelled fine. Well, when I took the paper off, she almost fell into my lap.

Glycolic or Alphahydroxy Acids

Later on, you'll be learning about the fruity glycolic acid peels (also called alphahydroxy acid peels) that physicians use in professional skin resurfacing techniques. These same acids (not as strongly formulated) are mixed into cleansers, astringents, creams, lotions, and gels and are available at discount drugstores without a prescription. For the first time, nonprescription skin-care products have an active ingredient that really works. Seven years ago, virtually no one had ever heard of glycolic acid, but this year, sales of products containing glycolic acid are expected to be over $1 billion.

The outer layer of your epidermis, as mentioned earlier, is always composed of dead cells. The skin works twenty-four hours a day (have you ever thought to thank your skin for its hard work?) to replace these dead cells as they are naturally shed. But as we age, this process slows down and becomes less efficient. Glycolic acid and other members of this family of chemicals such as lactic acid (the acid produced when milk sours) and pyruvic acid make skin look better by helping aged skin exfoliate more efficiently. It is the increased exfoliation that is responsible for the lovely effects these products can have on your complexion. There is some possibility that these products even may reverse some previous sun damage, but this is not known for sure.

These products can be applied as part of a regular facial routine very inexpensively, but you have to be patient, since it takes at least three to six months to see the benefit. Rough skin will be smoother, fine wrinkles will improve, and the skin will have a lovely, healthy glow. Another fine effect of glycolic acid is that it will help mild acne by opening up blocked pores. If you don't buy these products at expensive boutiques, but stick to discount drugstores, you will get a great value. Over-the-counter glycolic products are usually limited to strengths of 10 percent or less, which is enough for most people. If you want strengths of up to 20 percent for more effect, you can get a prescription through a dermatologist or cosmetic surgeon.

As you can tell, I think glycolic acid really works, and it does so with almost no side effects, but there are limitations. It won't do anything for moderate-to-deep wrinkles or scars. (For these kinds of problems, turn to chapter 7, "Skin Resurfacing," to learn about the latest in professional glycolic acid use and the carbon dioxide laser technique.) If your acne is any more serious than an occasional blocked pore, you need to be under the care of a dermatologist.

Retin-A

Retin-A (which is vitamin A acid, or tretinoin) is a very valuable prescription cream for treating acne. About ten years ago, many of my patients began to call me for refills of their retin-A far more often than usual, and it perplexed me. I called many of them to make sure they weren't wasting it by applying it too thickly, and still the refill calls were coming in at warp nine speed. After six months of this, there was the bombshell media announcement that retin-A actually could reduce wrinkles and rejuvenate the skin. No wonder parents were competing with their kids over the use of this very good product. I don't know who was the first person to realize that this wonderful unexpected benefit could come from an acne remedy, but doctors like me seem to have been the last to know that retin-A could help rejuvenate skin.

Retin-A improves the look of the skin by smoothing and thickening the outside layer and, like glycolic acid, it may repair previous sun damage to the skin. As with glycolic acid, you need to be patient to see the benefit, which again takes around three months to be noticeable. The skin will be smoother, softer, with less mottling and liver spots; fine wrinkles will diminish; and there'll be a more youthful, rosy color.

Johnson & Johnson's patent on retin-A is just about to run out, and when this happens, any pharmaceutical company will be able to produce generic, very inexpensive versions of it. To combat the likely loss of a great source of revenue, J&J came up with a slightly less irritating variation on the formula of retin-A. They are calling the new product Renova in the hopes that people will continue to buy their much more expensive name brand. For people to continue to spend more for the name brand, they will have to believe that Renova is better than both retin-A and the generic brands that will surely hit the marketplace after J&J's patent expires. My patients tell me that they see little, if any difference in the antiwrinkle effect of these two, and I am sure going to buy the generic brand for myself.

The major drawback is that retin-A can be very irritating, so you should start off with a low-strength .01 percent gel before increasing the concentration, as tolerated, to .025 percent cream. Many think that the redness and irritation that mark retin-A overuse are a sign that it is working. Well, if your goal is to have your facial skin feel like the sole of a shoe, you're on the right track. Better to only use retin-A if the previous use caused no irritation at all. Retin-A should only be applied at night, and you'll need to be especially certain to apply sun lotion during the day because it can aggravate the natural damage sun would cause. Most of my patients use glycolic acid during the day and retin-A at bedtime. It is my experience that, for most people, glycolic works better.

Coming Up Next:
Antioxidants and Betahydroxies

The latest wrinkle in the war against aging skin is an exciting class of chemicals called antioxidants. Basically, when cells are injured, oxygen free-radicals (or superoxides) are released that do further damage and impede healing. Exposure to that old villain, the ultraviolet radiation of the sun, is one of the chief ways for this damage to occur in the skin. The skin has antioxidants available to oppose this damage, but there aren't enough of them and they are easily exhausted. The idea here is to apply creams to the skin containing antioxidants such as vitamin C to replenish the body's supply of the damage-fighting chemicals. Vitamin C, in particular, is known to be a very potent antioxidant, as is glycolic acid and possibly even vitamin E.

Vitamin C is thought to actually protect the skin from the sun, but not enough to do so without also using sun protection. In fact, it's extremely important to understand that the antioxidant creams are not sunscreens, and if you're using them, you must protect your skin from the sun's rays just as you would (or should) do normally.

Products are popping up almost daily containing antioxidant ingredients and are being applied to the skin in every way imaginable, including by direct injection. To date, however, none of these treatments have been proven any more effective than plain moisturizers. Only time will tell if the antioxidants really fulfill their promise. Even if the theory behind them turns out to be valid, the overall effect antioxidants will have on the appearance of the skin will not be great and should, at best, be thought of as one of the many ways to improve the look of your skin.

Betahydroxies are very new, and similar to the glycolics in that they improve skin appearance by increasing exfoliation in the worn-out top layer of the epidermis. One of these, salicylic acid, is one of the most venerated and ancient of dermatological preparations. Found in the bark of willow trees, the Romans used it two thousand years ago to treat many conditions of the skin involving accumulation of dead cells, such as corns and calluses. In the last one hundred years, in more modern formulations, salicylic acid has been used very effectively to treat even dandruff, psoriasis, and warts.

As you now know, when we age, the natural exfoliation (shedding of the dead cells on the outside of the skin) decreases. The dead cells then accumulate, causing the skin to be drier, feel rough, and have an uneven texture. Some believe that the decrease in exfoliation may also be partly responsible for the finer wrinkles in our skin. By increasing exfoliation, both salicylic acid and the alphahydroxy acids cause these dead cells to be shed more efficiently, and over several months, the skin will become softer, smoother, and even have a better color and texture.

One of the things patients tell me really bothers them is that their pores get larger and darker with age. We dermatologists know that the main reason for this is that the dead cells and debris normally shed from skin gets stuck in the open pores, and this debris is very hard to remove. Salicylic acid is much more effective than glycolic and the other alphahydroxies in removing the debris from pores and will actually lighten them and make them appear smaller. Liver spots will also improve and the skin can develop a lovely, healthy glow. In general, salicylic acid preparations are much less irritating for most people than glycolic acid preparations and have less of a stinging burn when applied.

A Note of Caution

The antioxidants, alpha- and betahydroxy acids, and retin-A are collectively coming to be known as the bioactives. Scientific studies show that they can improve the appearance and feel of aging skin. Under no circumstances can they remotely improve moderate to deep wrinkles, and they are certainly no elixir of youth for the skin of the face, no matter how inflated, misleading, or false the claims of the manufacturers. Manufacturers have always added "new," "better" ingredients to products they wish to hawk to you, the consumer, and now some manufacturers are putting all these ingredients together as a kind of goulash in a single preparation to get you to buy it. No one knows whether these products can be mixed together harmoniously or whether the effect of one ingredient cancels out the effect of others because they should not be combined. You need to remember that currently the government is not regulating these new products in any meaningful way, and at the same time, you should stay tuned. These new acids are arriving so quickly that, by the time you read this, a new "do it yourself" formula may be hitting the market. Be cautious, but be informed—I doubt there's any more important advice a doctor could give to a medical consumer.

FREQUENTLY ASKED QUESTIONS

Can't I make wrinkles go away with the right exercise?

The notion that exercising the facial muscles can strengthen them in a way that will tighten and lift the face is worthy of P. T. Barnum. I have never met anyone for whom it worked, no matter how long they practiced, but it's a myth that just won't die.

Just this past year in fact there was a springlike device being sold nationally that fit into the mouth that proved to be very popular. I saw a demonstration of it on television one night, and watching the crazy faces made by the people doing these exercises in the infomercial . . . well, I could only think that this must be how Jim Carrey got his start in show business. There was also a bestselling book, *Facercize*, which taught you another set of ex-exercises to try—maybe for the people who were disappointed that the spring didn't seem to be doing enough.

Honestly, save your money. Facial exercises in cosmetic surgery are best done when your surgeon quotes you the fees for the procedures.

Does smoking really cause wrinkles?

I'm sure you'll be shocked to hear me say that smoking is terrible for the skin. The worst wrinkles I have ever seen on the face, especially around the lips, occur in long-term smokers. The constant pursing of the lips grooves these wrinkles into the skin as if they were made by a woodworker's awl, and the smoke itself touching the skin vastly speeds up its aging and may in fact directly cause the skin to develop a cancer. Smoking keeps down the amount of oxygen circulating in your bloodstream, and since the skin is rich in blood vessels, smoking is basically a method of starving your face.

I almost never do a facelift on a smoker unless he or she stops well before the surgery, because smoking in the immediate post-operative period can so decrease the blood supply to the healing skin that huge patches may be lost, leading to horrendous scarring and deformity. So, if the prospects of emphysema and lung cancer aren't enough to turn you away from coffin nails, perhaps not being allowed your God-given right to a facelift will make you strive harder to quit. I certainly hope so.

What is the difference between a $10 moisturizer and a $40 one?

Thirty dollars (drum roll). I mean this. All well-made moisturizers are the same to the skin. The skin doesn't appreciate or know when you have spent money on a high-end product that does nothing different than the inexpensive one. Save your money.

What are the signs of skin cancer?

More than 500,000 Americans a year are diagnosed with skin cancer, representing an explosive growth over the past three decades. The vast majority of these cases are directly related to unprotected sun exposure.

Any spot on the skin that's new, or, more commonly, an old spot that changes, should be evaluated by a dermatologist if it doesn't go away completely by itself after several weeks. Changes include the color lightening or darkening; the size increasing or shrinking; the border going from smooth to irregular; itching; or a patch of damaged skin that won't heal. Yes, there's a lot of latitude in these categories, but that's because only a trained dermatologist or pathologist can diagnose skin cancer correctly, and if any of these signs are present, you should see your doctor immediately. Don't wait, delay, or try to diagnose yourself.

The most deadly form of skin cancer is malignant melanoma, or mole cancer. When a mole turns malignant, or more rarely when a malignant mole arises on what was unmarked skin, quick intervention is the answer, and it may well save your life. Roughly one American dies every hour from mole cancer. So if any of these signs appear, don't try to be your own doctor and don't delay. The vast majority of those who have died of skin cancer might have been saved if they'd been treated in time. It takes only moments and usually leaves no scar whatsoever for a dermatologist to biopsy a suspicious mole that a pathologist can then check under a microscope. And, if caught in time, a skin cancer can be cured immediately by removing the malignancy.

Almost twenty years ago, I got a letter from a man who heard me talking about mole cancer on the radio and went immediately to a dermatologist. He had been worried for several months about a growth on his back, which turned out to be a malignant melanoma. There is no question in this man's mind— or mine—that any further delay could have been fatal.

Chapter 3

HOW TO CHOOSE
A DOCTOR

THE POLITICS OF
LOOKING YOUR BEST;
THE CONSULTATION;
ANESTHESIA TODAY

et's say you've now considered the various issues, looked carefully at yourself, spent some time going over your feelings, and are ready to move forward. After reviewing the list of problems and procedures in the introduction and after reading the appropriate chapters, you know pretty much what kind of cosmetic procedure to consider, and now you need to find a doctor who specializes in the work you require and has a temperament and a style that fit you.

Unfortunately, this isn't easy; it will take effort on your part to find just the right surgeon. You need to become educated about the field and do plenty of comparison shopping. It would be much easier if it were a simple matter of schooling, degrees, and medical specialty, but cosmetic surgery is about on-the-job training. The right surgeon for you will be the one who has done the procedure you want numerous times on people with features similar to yours and who has successfully gotten the results you're hoping to achieve.

One of my patients, Jayne, told me:

I was unhappy and dissastisfied with the results I was getting at the gym, even though I worked out four times a week. I finally decided I'd get liposuction, and spent a lot of time looking for the right doctor, talking to friends, my personal doctors, reading every article I could so I'd be intelligent enough to ask the right questions. I interviewed three cosmetic surgeons, and it was obvious that one really had the expertise. He was up front and never vague about what would happen; he told me exactly what I could and couldn't expect.

You can just tell when someone's done something so many times that your case is nothing they haven't seen before, so there won't be any surprises coming up. After all, if anybody was going to touch my body, it was going to be someone who really knew what they were doing.

The Politics of Looking Your Best

Wading through the various medical specialties is one of the most confusing issues for anyone looking for a surgeon. Cosmetic surgeon, plastic surgeon, reconstructive surgeon, dermatological surgeon, ENT (ear, nose, and throat) surgeon, eye surgeon— these terms are so bewildering that even I can get as confused as Costello in the Abbott and Costello routine "Who's on first."

Doctors are just like you in that they take pride in their work and want to do what they have studied and been trained to do, which, in the case of cosmetic surgery, is to make people look and feel their best. In a perfect and civilized world, doctors would share their expertise and techniques openly with all like-minded doctors, even those in different areas of specialization, and in fact many do. But in the real world of too many doctors and a multitude of specialties, each specialist is convinced he or she should perform your surgery, and doctors sometimes act more like warriors in hostile tribes than like brothers and sisters in a fraternity of healing. When looking for the most qualified doctor to do your surgery, look beyond labels, titles, and the skirmishes of the warring tribes before deciding who will win you and your hard-earned dollars. My experience is that the more doctors talk about credentials, training, and titles, the more they are really concerned about turf and money.

I am a cosmetic surgeon, by which I mean that my whole career is solely directed toward making people look their best, and I do no reconstructive work at all. So even though I've been trained to do skin grafting and to remove cancers, and I have the knowledge to perform many other reconstructive techniques for those who've had accidents or disfiguring birth defects, I've spent more than twenty years making aesthetic improvements. This is a key point. *Aesthetic* and *reconstructive* surgeries are not the same; they require a different mindset on the part of the surgeon.

To add to the confusion, many people think plastic surgery is synonymous with aesthetic surgery, when just the opposite is true. As the *Encyclopaedia Britannica* puts it: "The term *plastic* refers to the molding and reshaping of body tissues—bone, fat, muscle, cartilage, and skin." Pure plastic surgery is reconstructive in nature and has as its goal repairing injuries such as burns or correcting birth defects such as cleft palates, to name just a few. A great plastic surgeon needs to have a terrific aesthetic sense so that the repairs produce the most visually pleasing result, but enhancing appearance in otherwise healthy people is not the primary goal of pure plastic surgery. Keep in mind that the vast majority of nose jobs, facelifts, and breast surgeries are done on perfectly healthy people who want to look their best, and this falls into the category that I call aesthetic surgery. Though many doctors can do both aesthetic and reconstructive surgery with great skill, I personally always look for the specialist.

Alan's Doctor-Finder Rule 1: When you look for a cosmetic surgeon, try to find a specialist who primarily does aesthetic work, no matter what his or her specialty. There are so many to choose from that this shouldn't be a tough criterion.

I am also a board-certified dermatologist. You may ask, Aren't dermatologists the doctors who treat your kid's acne, itchy toes, and the heartbreak of psoriasis? Yes we are, but dermatology as a specialty has also been a key specialty for research and development in cosmetic surgery—as has plastic surgery, ENT surgery, eye surgery, and the field of cosmetology. For example, here are just some of the major advancements we "derms" have contributed to the field:

- *Face peel* (1882): Dr. Unna brings the recipes to America for phenol and TCA peels, recipes originating from German gypsies who passed them on through the centuries.
- *Dermabrasion* (1952): Dr. Abner Kurtin reports his technique, including the use of instruments similar to the ones used today.
- *Hair transplant* (1959): Dr. Norman Orentreich reports the first successful technique for male pattern hair loss.
- *Laser surgery* (1961): Dr. Leon Goldman becomes the first physician to apply laser methods to human medical needs, becoming the father of all laser surgery used in all medical specialties.
- *Liposuction* (1977): Dr. Lawrence Field is one of the first American doctors to learn and introduce Dr. Gerard Illouz's techniques in the United States.
- *Collagen injections* (1979): Dr. Arnold Klein pioneers the use of collagen from lab work done at Stanford University.
- *Tumescent liposuction* (1987): Dr. Jeff Klein publishes his landmark paper on methods of removing fat more safely and with more precision than ever before, a technique still in use today.
- *Laser skin resurfacing with carbon dioxide, retin-A, and glycolic acid* (1980s and 1990s): These treatments owe their birth and advancement to dermatologists such as Dr. Larry David, Dr. Al Kligman, and Dr. Van Scott.

Of course, dermatology was not alone in contributing to the evolution of cosmetic surgery. Plastic surgery was fundamentally responsible for inventing and developing crucial procedures such as the facelift, browlift, tummy tuck, and all forms of aesthetic breast surgery. Some of the earliest writings on nose enhancement (rhinoplasty) are in ENT literature, and ophthalmologists fundamentally developed aesthetic eye surgery.

But which specialty should be given exact credit for which procedure is not completely clear. As I've shown, many procedures we think of as modern, such as the face peel, dermabrasion, and skin grafting, really began thousands of years ago and were practiced by lay people who would hardly be considered health professionals. Where does the "invented by" credit really go if Cleopatra used peels that are nearly identical to those in popular use today?

It's common today for a medical specialty to invent or advance a technique that another specialty will adopt as its own, often adding greatly to the effectiveness and benefit. A good example of this is the phenol face peel: Dr. Unna, a dermatologist, brought the formula to America more than one hundred years ago, but it is Drs. Thomas Baker and Howard Gordon, plastic surgeons, who changed the recipe and made the phenol peel a reliable and safe modality to retexture aged facial skin. No matter which specialty invents a new procedure, over time the procedure will cross over to other specialties that will change and improve the procedure.

Problems occur when a specialty develops or expropriates a technique and, human nature being what it is, some members of that specialty feel that they should do that technique to the exclusion of all others. Richard Webster, M.D., a great plastic surgeon and teacher who freely shared his techniques with earnest student doctors of all stripes, wrote the following in the introduction to a cosmetic surgery textbook:

> A common pattern of behavior seems to exist here. Those who believe that they have established "ownership rights" in a given field of human endeavor organize to provide a forum for discussion and education of those in a given field. Generally, they organize also to protect the egos, power, and economic endeavors of those in their organization. A vested interest in maintenance

of the status quo seems to develop in what is considered "their field." It is human and natural for a group to behave in this fashion; it is only at an intellectual level that certain individuals in a given field can force themselves to behave in the long term interests of human progress and the public good, to share ego satisfaction, power, and economic benefits with those from other groups whose work overlaps that of the already organized group.

It is crucial to honor the pioneers, leaders, and mavericks who had the vision, foresight, and courage to invent new techniques that have made cosmetic surgery the wonderful medical endeavor it is. But, as you now know, once techniques are out there, they are picked up by all the other medical specialties who have similar interests. Sometimes a patient who consults with me will say that their eye doctor (ophthalmologist) wants to do their eyelid lift. Another patient who comes to see me about liposuction will tell me that their gynecologist wants to do their lipo. These people ask me what I think. I firmly believe that any cosmetic surgeon from any specialty can do the work if he or she is well trained, experienced, and specializes in that particular procedure. In all the years I spent in the dermatology departments at Yale University and the University of Califonia, San Francisco, I personally never saw a single hair transplant, dermabrasion, or aesthetic face peel. Patients are always amazed when I tell them this at consultations. How can this be? Didn't dermatologists invent these techniques?

The great American medical teaching schools and hospitals are geared toward research and reconstructive surgery. Cosmetic surgery is usually not emphasized; there are few, if any, professors of cosmetic surgery; and in general, cosmetic or aesthetic surgery is regarded as a less important, lower calling because it is about beauty, not biological function. In my era of training, very few student dermatologists, plastic surgeons, or ENTs ever saw any aesthetic surgery during their years of formal residency instruction. Though this has changed somewhat in the last few years, the emphasis in the university is not on cosmetic surgery. Those of us who exclusively do cosmetic surgery have in the past, and will continue in the present, to do our most important training after we have finished our formal hospital work. We train in cosmetic surgery by taking specialized fellowships, by going to specialized, professional meetings and training with the masters and leaders in the field from many different specialties.

Alan's Doctor-Finder Rule 2: Beware the use of titles and diplomas as your exclusive guide to choosing the right doctor. It's not the paper—it's the practice! If a doctor has successfully performed the surgery you want many, many times, it doesn't matter what degree he or she attained two decades ago. I have wonderful diplomas from Yale and the University of California on my wall, but that isn't why I do wonderful cosmetic surgery. It is the training and help I have had and continue to have over the years from the greatest teachers and mentors in the world that has made me what I am.

I've written this section to show the rich heritage and complex tapestry of the specialty we call cosmetic surgery and to show that it belongs to no one medical specialty, interest group, or organization but to all well-trained physicians who have spent the time and effort to practice their craft with skill, safety, and loving attention to the wants and needs of their patients.

The Consultation

You've now gotten a list of prospective surgeons, either from friends, other doctors, maybe even a local hospital or medical association. The next step is to make appointments with each for a consultation, and if you're nervous about taking this step, don't feel alone. A consultation in cosmetic surgery is just like a cross between test driving a car and going on a blind date. Both parties are expectant, a little nervous, on their best behavior, and trying to figure out if they should have a second date—in this case, go ahead with elective surgery (or at least return for a second consultation). You, the consumer, should know what to expect, what to ask, what to look out for, and the important questions you need to have answered before you leave. Remember, you should go back for a second consultation or at least call and have additional questions answered if anything is unclear; then, after all your medical questions have been fully answered, take your time, speak to people who have your best interests at heart, and listen to your inner self before making a final decision.

THE DOCTOR'S OFFICE

Cosmetic surgeons usually have elegant offices with great attention to details, like color and fabric, that will convey to patients a feeling of safety, comfort, and beauty. This is the norm in this specialty, so don't be put off by Oriental rugs, expensive wall art, beautiful views or sculptures, and a general air of success. Most cosmetic surgeons decorate their offices this way because: they think the patients expect it; they worry that the competitive surgeon down the hall may have a prettier office; and most surgeons believe that potential patients may subtly feel a beautiful, tasteful working environment is a reflection of the doctor's ability to do consistently beautiful work.

If the office has neon glow colors that are mismatched, clashing wall coverings and rugs, and gives the impression that the doctor is colorblind, would you really want that person to do your facelift? More important than the look of the office, however, is the behavior of the staff. Are they friendly, helpful, and pleasant or superior, intimidating, and distant? You can learn a great deal about whether or not a doctor is right for you by his or her staff and office environment.

THE INTERVIEW

The actual meeting with the doctor and staff occurs on several different levels beyond the passing back and forth of factual information you need to know to be able to make an informed decision. It's best for you to start off by telling the doctor what bothers you. If, before you can even open your mouth, the doctor gives you a long list of your cosmetic deficiencies and a $15,000 plan to correct them, this is a bad beginning. I firmly believe that the only procedures that should be discussed are those that will solve problems important to and put forward by the patient.

Now is when you have to get down to the nitty-gritty and discuss in great detail, with a doctor you've just met, that part of your appearance that bothers you the most. No one really wants to do this, of course, but if your potential surgeon has any experience and understanding at all, he or she should be able to put you at ease rapidly. If you get the feeling the doctor hasn't seen problems similar to yours many times before, you're probably at the wrong office. Your doctor will probably take photographs of problem areas you have spent most of your life trying to from others. Just keep in mind that this is the beginning of changing yourself for the better.

After you've told the doctor what bothers you and what you'd like to accomplish, there should be a thorough discussion of what the procedure you need entails. All information should be given to you in plain, simple English. The basics of all these techniques are not complicated, and you should understand how the procedure you are inquiring about works; how it can work for you personally; how to prepare yourself beforehand; how long the surgery will actually take; whether you are going home afterward or staying in the facility overnight; when you should expect to see the benefits of your surgery; and, most important, the potential risks versus the benefits of going ahead. This should take, minimally, thirty to sixty minutes.

You should always see before-and-after pictures of people with problems similar to yours; in fact, you should spend some time looking at many pictures of patients similar to you (skin tone, age, body type, and facial type) who had the same type of condition, so as to get a real feel for the doctor's quality and breadth of work. I've often heard patients who consult with me say that another physician they visited did not want to show them before-and-after photos because then the patient would expect exactly that result. All surgeons should be proud to show examples of their best work, and for a doctor to say this to you speaks very poorly of their trust in your intelligence. Patients know and can be told that a before-and-after picture shows one possible outcome and not the exact one they will get.

Some doctors use computer imaging; they take a picture of you, project it onto the computer screen, and then use a mouse to change your face or body to show you the results. I tried this several years ago, but it created confusion, as clients thought they would get the exact same result they had seen on the screen. This could never be true since we all heal differently and each of us will get slightly different results, even if the surgeon were to do, like a robot, precisely the same technique on everyone. Because of this confusion, doctors using computer imaging had to get clients to sign a legal release after seeing the computer-generated results saying they knew the actual outcome of their surgeries would not be identical to the simulation.

You may want to ask the doctor for the phone numbers of patients who've had the same work that you're considering and give them a call. If the doctor says he or she can't or won't give out phone numbers, that's a major warning sign. You can also get a feel about others' experiences by showing up early or staying late after your appointment and chatting with others in the waiting room. See what their experiences have been and judge for yourself.

Finally, the doctor should ask if you have questions, and, if you do, all your questions should be answered before you leave. A reluctance on the part of the doctor to answer questions is not acceptable and is another possible warning sign that you are in the wrong office. Patients are often embarrassed or worried about asking what they think are silly or stupid questions. I have never heard a question that is silly or stupid. You are there, after all, to be informed about matters that are outside your expertise. You should have a prepared set of questions written down before you arrive and, most important, you should ask *any* questions you have, no matter how foolish or minor they may seem. The elective surgery patient can never be too informed. You consider many brands when shopping for a dishwasher, or a car, or a home computer; I recommend you consult with at least three doctors before selecting a cosmetic surgeon.

THE CRUCIAL QUESTIONS YOU SHOULD ASK

Whenever I go to a restaurant that has a huge menu, I always think: The chef can't be great at making all these dishes and I wish I could know what the chef specializes in or really loves to cook. I feel this applies to cosmetic surgery as well. There are many superbly trained surgeons who consistently have wonderful results doing a large variety of procedures, but when I think back over the last twenty years to my own great teachers and mentors, they all had small menus.

You can find out if this is the right doctor for you by asking:

Where did the doctor train?

Most of us first learn to do procedures in officially sanctioned courses where teachers are leaders in the field and give formal lectures on technique. Usually the student will then get a certificate attesting to attendance. Whether the student actually attended the lectures (or was out at the pool or golf course when the lecture was given) will not be on the certificate. In my experience, the vast majority of doctors do attend lectures and want to learn all that they can. At these meetings sometimes videos or even live demonstrations of surgery are presented, which is better than lectures. Such demonstrations show doctors how the surgery is actually performed. Doctors usually present their certificates of attendance to their medical insurance companies before actually attempting the procedure in question for the first time. Though this system is time-honored and in use today, there is an additional step that can even better prepare your doctor to begin a new technique.

Who did the doctor train with?

The best training I have ever had was when I visited the actual clinics of the greatest pioneers and practitioners of techniques. This process called mentoring or preceptorship. No other form of medical education can top actually watching the hands of a great surgeon. Students can see great work, know what to aspire to, and learn the art before having to do it on their own.

Watching Dr. Yves Gerard Illouz, one of the inventors of liposuction, actually operate in Paris on three separate trips, or visiting Dr. O'tar Norwood, a great hair transplant surgeon in Oklahoma City, or seeing Dr. Luiz Toledo in São Paulo, Brazil, actually do liposculpture have easily been among the greatest and most useful experiences in my professional life. Sometimes I've even had a master surgeon come to my clinic and observe me doing surgery to ensure I have fully grasped their technique. It is wonderful to be able to ask them questions in situ and learn from their experiences.

How often does the doctor perform that surgery?

Doctors are like all of us: They do best what they do most often. If you ask your potential surgeon how often he or she performs, for example, laser eyelid lifts and the response is a long pause or if the doctor calls in the chief scrub nurse to ask where the instruments were put after the last surgery and there is another pause . . . this is not my idea of specialization.

It is true that surgeons do fine work with procedures they don't do very often, but when looking for a doctor for myself or my family, I look for a long and large experience based on repeated success with the same surgery. How often is enough? There is no exact answer to this question, but certainly at least several times per month.

How many procedures has the doctor done?

There is really some safety in numbers. A physician who has done three hundred facelifts has got to be more comfortable in the technique than one who has done fifty. However, this only goes so far, because there are some very poorly trained doctors who never do good work in spite of endless trying year after year. This is the kind of "practice" you don't want from your doctor.

Some beginners who are gifted and exquisitely trained can do great work from the start, and, like anyone, doctors can fib or bend the truth. A typical example would be for a doctor to tell a patient he or she has done five hundred liposuctions, when what is really meant is that he or she has done ten body areas (two hips, two saddlebags, two knees, two ankles, one stomach, and one neck) on fifty people. So, at your consultation, be specific and ask the doctor how many clients he or she has had for your particular procedure.

What are the actual complications the doctor's other patients have had with this surgery?

Cosmetic surgery can have tragic complications, some leading to loss of life. Every doctor has had patients who have developed complications and should be completely candid with you about what happened.

I think patients seldom listen really closely when potential risks, such as infection and scarring, are explained, thinking these happen only to someone else. When the doctor levels with the patient and talks about actual infections or injuries that have occurred with real people, then the possibility becomes real and concrete.

There is absolutely no one answer as to how many complications should make you wary about staying with the doctor you're interviewing. Your choice, of course, also depends on the number of years the doctor has been in practice and how many cases he or she sees in a week. After listening to the possible complications and asking questions about them, however, you should have a real feeling about whether your doctor is candid, forthright, trustworthy, and within your comfort zone of safety.

ON A DEEPER LEVEL

As you now know, consults work on several levels, just like blind dates. You should use your own sixth sense to determine whether the doctor is comfortable not only with explaining the information to you, but also with the information itself. You will know long before you leave the office whether the doctor actually has confidence in his or her ability to do that surgery. I said confidence, not brashness or arrogance. Anyone who loves their work and is good at it should positively glow when explaining it. If other staff members are present, you can observe how the doctor interacts with them—is their attitude genuinely respectful? Attila the Hun probably could have been trained to do liposuction, but would you have wanted to go to him?

One key item that few patients observe is that, during a consultation, the doctor is also carefully looking you over. One of my own professional stoplights during this process is people who see the world as totally black or white and want all-or-nothing results. Unfortunately, cosmetic surgery (like marriage, parenting, or the stock market, to name just a few examples) doesn't work that way. People can achieve great improvement with a skillful cosmetic surgeon, but we cannot make a human being over again or achieve an absolutely perfect result every time. So as soon as I hear a patient ask for perfection, I know I will never operate on them, simply because they will never be happy. Aspiring to perfection is one thing, but demanding and being unwilling to settle for less is another.

My operations director, Magda Rodrigues, has performed many consults and is immensely popular with my patients for her direct, down-to-earth nature. She feels one of the biggest problems in consults is when someone says they want something "fixed" or "cured." In that situation, Magda always firmly replies that cosmetic surgery can improve or make a problem better but cannot "fix" or "cure" it. If a person at a consult keeps referring to "fixes," she knows this is someone who is not going to be satisfied with the results that aesthetic surgery can achieve.

I like hearing patients ask for improvement; I can always work with that person. My patients and I spend at least six months together after surgery following their progress. It is important for me to work with patients who have expectations that I can deliver, but I also prefer working with people who love themselves as they are and think life is pretty good—except for those droopy eyelids, oversized hips, or deep wrinkles.

Cosmetic surgery, in fact, works best on people who are relatively content in life, who like themselves the way they are. When people come into the office and I hear them hoping surgery will make them better people or that it will make them more popular, or if I can tell that the person does not like him or herself, every alarm bell in my being goes off. People can only love and respect themselves from within. No surgeon, indeed no other person, can give that from without. On the other hand, losing a droopy eyelid or, after lipo, slipping into slinky, tight clothes, may be just the confidence boost that allows a patient to enjoy more energy and success in life.

After you have a chance to meet with various candidates for the job, sit back and let your mind consider all of the issues involved in making this decision. Who had the office environment you found most to your liking? Did any of the before pictures remind you of yourself, and did any of the afters show what you hoped your results might be? Return for a second consultation, but once you've made your choice, let the doctor you've selected know as soon as possible. Some of the more popular surgeons, obviously, are very busy, and you'll want to now create a schedule that suits both of you.

Anesthesia Today

In my practice, I've found that it's very common for patients to have more worries about the anesthesia than the surgery. You can rest assured, however, because in the past ten years there have been many wonderful advances in the science of eliminating pain. We now have drugs with rapid-onset metabolism and elimination, which means you get to go home sooner after surgery than ever before. Very few people today wake up from surgery with the nausea and hangover side-effects that were so common in the past. Breakthroughs in equipment (such as devices that measure the gasses in your breath) allow the anesthesiologist to monitor your well-being with tremendous accuracy, meaning greater safety for you. Additionally, there now are a variety of anesthesia techniques and we can sometimes offer patients their choice of general anesthesia (which makes you unconscious), intravenous sedation (sometimes called twilight anesthesia, which leaves you semi-awake), or regional anesthesia (which only affects a specific part of the body).

All the anesthesiologists in my clinic are board-certified physicians with specialized postdoctoral training. So, when you have surgery, you are actually being treated by two doctors at once. The surgeon deals directly with the body part to be repaired (or in the cosmetic surgeon's case, improved) while the anesthesiologist monitors your vital signs, including your cardiac status, respiration, temperature, state of consciousness, and feelings of pain. If any of these areas fall outside a healthy range, the anesthesiologist is the one who administers corrective fluids (including balanced salt and sugar solutions), as well as making adjustments to the anesthesia itself. Surgery involves real teamwork, so asking about the anesthesiologist during your consultation is important. You may even want to speak with him or her directly before making your choice of surgeons, which is in fact the recommendation of the American Society of Anesthesiologists. At the very least, it's very important for you to talk with the anesthesiologist several days ahead of surgery so he or she can know your medical history, whether you have any allergies to medications, and how you've responded to anesthesia in previous surgeries.

Some anesthesiologists are highly specialized. Ones who specialize in cosmetic surgery, such as those I work with, can do many things to help me do my best work. For example, in liposuction it's very important that the anesthesiologist replace some of the fluid that comes out with the removed fat with salt solutions, and when I do a laser eyelid lift, an anesthesiologist specializing in cosmetic surgery knows how to slightly lower the patient's blood pressure to decrease bleeding. With certain kinds of facelifts, the patient must lie very still, so the anesthesiologist will administer relaxing sedatives to make holding still something that feels easy and natural to do.

QUESTIONS TO ASK DURING THE CONSULTATION

Is the anesthesia administered by a board-certified anesthesiologist? Is he or she particularly experienced with (if not a specialist in) cosmetic surgery? Will he or she be in the office the whole day to monitor you until you go home?

In case anything goes the slightest bit wrong, having both doctors available on-site is always the best choice.

Will there be a registered nurse specifically trained and experienced in recovery care to look after you postoperatively?

Another assurance of safety and always preferred.

Is the office certified by a regulatory agency?

In many states (such as California), all outpatient clinics that perform surgery must go through a certification process.

FREQUENTLY ASKED QUESTIONS

Will I be awake during the procedure or completely knocked out?

For most procedures, you can decide on your level of alertness. Full body liposuction, for example, can be done under regional or general anesthesia.

"I'm worried about the anesthesia because the last time I had surgery, it made me sick."

The new drugs don't cause anywhere near the nausea and other side-effects that once occurred so frequently, and we now have many treatments to combat these kinds of problems if they do occur.

Part Two

THE PROCEDURES

*

Chapter 4

TIGHTENING THE TURKEY NECK

A REVOLUTIONARY NEW TECHNIQUE TO FIX DROOP AND WATTLES

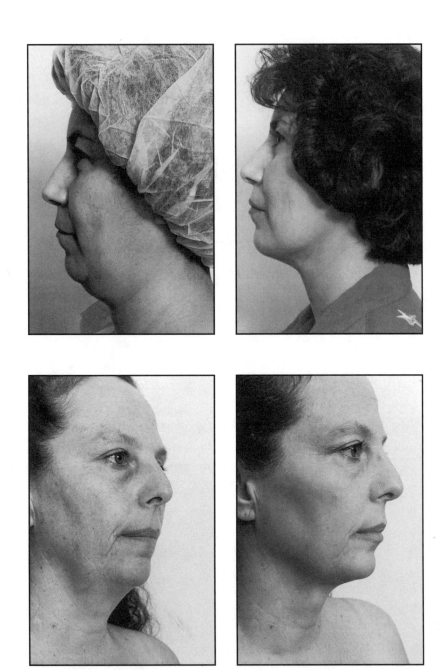

Neck Microsuctions—before and after

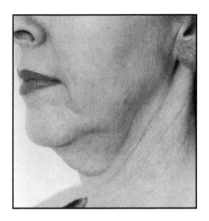 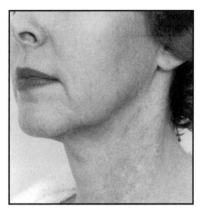

As we age, many of us develop droopy "turkey" necks, and this condition is so common that the fashion industry has developed a whole area of expertise in covering up the necks of older men and women. For decades, the only improvement a cosmetic surgeon could offer was the classic lower facelift, but you only have to watch the Academy Awards and see all the aged Hollywood stars (who've been pulled so tight they look like they've got their heads out the window of an airborne 747) to understand why so many of the turkey neck–afflicted would never even consider having a lower lift.

At its best, a lower facelift can improve and rejuvenate the face, but even then, facelifts frequently involve highly visible scars behind the ears, a long recovery time, and great expense and inconvenience. Additionally, for many people, the benefits of a lower facelift will begin to fade after a year or two, and this seems to me an incredible rigmarole and expense to go to for such a short-term benefit. The speed of aging is never slowed by having a cosmetic surgery procedure, so if a first facelift creates a mild wind-tunnel look, the second or third lift may produce the look of a permanent leer.

I first realized that there was a genuine alternative to this state of affairs when, in 1990, I visited Dr. Luiz Toledo, the great São Paulo surgeon, to observe as he treated patients with loose, wrinkly skin under their chins. The trip began because my entire staff is always on the lookout for new ideas and techniques in cosmetic surgery, and my Brazilian-born ops director, Magda Rodrigues (then my nurse), came in with *Manchete,* a Brazilian magazine, to show me an article on the now world-famous Dr. Toledo. What he was doing, according to this article, was so astonishing that I was sure it was a hoax, but Magda insisted it must be true, and so the two of us flew down to Brazil.

In the operating room we watched as Dr. Toledo used a modified fat removal technique that was so revolutionary, offbeat, and beyond my initial comprehension that, being an ex–New Yorker, I couldn't believe my eyes. I watched him numb the patient's neck with a little local anesthetic (Lidocaine) and then use a small blunt rod to remove the fat. As he was doing this, he told me, with a completely straight face, that over the following four to six months, the skin would actually tighten and tuck under the chin like wallpaper.

Now let me digress for a moment and tell you why, at that time, I didn't believe a word of it. One of the most fundamental ABCs of liposuction is that you never try to treat skin that is loose. A classic example of this would be in a man who has gained and lost weight many times, or a woman who has had children and, because of the weight gain from pregnancy, has been left with permanent loose stomach skin. The belief has always been that, because the underlying fat is actually supporting that worn-out skin, removing it will leave the skin even looser than it was before, which is about as bad a mistake as you can make in lipo.

So I'm watching Dr. Toledo do this fat removal procedure on people with very loose neck skin in 1990, and I'm smugly thinking to myself that he doesn't know as much about lipo as I do, and I'm certain that the results will be disastrous. In fact, at the end of the first morning, all I could think was how I could gracefully get out of his clinic to do a little sightseeing before heading home. I didn't, of course, since that would have been an insult to Dr. Toledo, but I was certain this whole trip had been a waste of time.

I got back to my practice in San Francisco, two months went by, when a package from Dr. Toledo arrived with photos of the results. Looking at these before-and-afters of people who we'd seen directly was like one of those amazing moments where time seems to stop and you realize that something momentous has happened and that your life will never be the same again. It wasn't exactly the wonderful feeling of joy and awe that I'd had when my children were born, but it was really close. Toledo's patients' necks were so much tighter than before that I knew I had failed to appreciate one of the greatest advances in cosmetic surgery I had ever witnessed. Needless to say, I immediately called my travel agent and took the next flight back to Brazil, genuinely humbled.

I've visited Dr. Toledo many times since, and over the years in my office I've reshaped the instruments and slowly improved his method to where it can even help people who are more than eighty years old. But the basic principles remain the same. I call this tightening of the turkey-neck skin without any skin removal *neck microsuction,* and the results are so amazing that, when I show patients before-and-after pictures of this technique, I usually get a look like I'm trying to sell them the Golden Gate Bridge for a buck. Their disbelief is only increased when I tell them the procedure is done outpatient and under local anesthetic, takes little more than an hour, and involves no skin removal and no suturing whatsoever.

We get loose neck skin from a lifetime of gravity pulling the skin down. In consults I like to use the analogy of a man's underwear having been washed so many times that the rubber waistband becomes hopelessly stretched out. If the fabric of the underwear is still good and you don't want to throw it away, you can do one of two things: You can snip out the extra rubber and sew the ends of the bands together until the waist is comfortably snug again, or you can put in an entirely new waistband. It doesn't take an Einstein to realize that the new waistband is the better approach and, in fact, will last a lot longer.

A classic lower facelift done at any level of skill is, for me, like mending the old waistband. No matter how much you stretch that old worn-out skin by pulling it behind the ears, the elastic rubber bands in the skin are still shot from gravity and will loosen again very quickly. On the other hand, my technique of neck microsuction really is the equivalent of threading brand-new rubber bands into the skin, and this may explain why, almost without exception, the people I performed neck micro-suction on eight years ago have not needed to repeat the proce-dure.

When one of my patients, Phyllis Kromer, turned sixty-eight, she decided to have a whole new life. She dieted and lost fifty-five pounds, which left her with what she called

a big ugly turkey neck that really bugged me. I am in wonderful health and feel great and I think I ought to look great, too. I have this boundless energy and wanted to look as fresh as I feel. We should all live by that Army motto: "Be all that you can be."

I did a lot of research and went to several cosmetic surgeons about this turkey neck, and they all wanted to do drastic surgery and that just didn't sit right with me. Then I heard about Dr. Gaynor and went on the Internet and saw all about his micro-suction technique. The surgery was a piece of cake; I told my husband I couldn't believe there was no pain. The recovery was so nothing that I didn't end up with a single scar.

The Preparation

A thorough history is taken at the consultation to make sure prospective patients are in good health. If they have underlying chronic conditions (such as diabetes, heart disease, or high blood pressure), it's almost never a problem for a cosmetic procedure as long as the illnesses are in good control and are being actively managed by a family doctor. When I am the slightest bit unsure, I call the family doctor to make sure the patient is properly following a medical regimen. A blood test is also required to check for anemia, blood abnormalities, or a hidden bleeding tendency. It is crucial the person be off aspirin, certain cold remedies, and alcohol, because these greatly increase the possibility of bleeding or severe bruising.

The Procedure

Neck microsuction is probably the most patient-friendly of all cosmetic surgeries. It's an outpatient procedure that takes little more than an hour and can be performed in a small procedure room. Patients wear a paper gown and a sterile drape, and most barely notice the anesthesia injections. I always say to patients, as I numb them, to tell me in their own terms how much it hurts, on a scale from one to ten, with ten being the pain level of having your appendix removed on the prairie without any anesthesia. The answer is almost always two or three, and once the neck is numb, there is no pain at all during the procedure.

After the skin of the neck is thoroughly cleansed with antiseptic solution, I numb a small area of the skin just under the chin and just behind and in back of the earlobes, hidden from view. Then I make a small entry through the skin, and through that entry I inject more local anesthetic until the whole neck has been treated. Next I wait for twenty to thirty minutes to allow the tissue to marinate. Surprisingly, the injecting of the local anesthetic is so relatively painless that more than half the patients do not want any form of mild sedation at all, and the other half just put a sedative pill such as Valium under their tongue. When the patient is ready I use a small, blunt, hollow tube, called a *cannula* (about one-eighth of an inch in diameter), attached to a small syringe, to remove all the extra fat from the neck. I begin by using the entry just under the chin and moving the rod back and forth gently, like the bowing of a violin. I next insert the rod into the entry behind each ear aiming toward the chin area from the side. The effect of this is to leave long, hollow tunnels in the fat, very much like the holes in Swiss cheese. The exact placement of these tunnels is critical, making neck microsuction what we call "technique dependent"; the surgeon has to know exactly what he or she is doing or the final result will be neither smooth nor symmetrical. The tunnels are made of all different sizes, at all different depths of the fat, and going in all different planned directions so that there are no drop-offs, steplike dips, or visible lines in the skin. When all goes well, the final result yields a wonderfully tighter neck with a seamless harmony between the affected areas and the surrounding untouched areas. Once the fat is removed, the skin tightening begins.

To tighten the skin, I insert another blunt, hollow, even narrower cannula that I use to scratch the underside of the skin (the dermis) through the three entry points. Because I use the syringe to apply gentle suction through the rod as I move back and forth, and the rod has narrow holes along its side, and the effect produced is like that of taking smooth Parmesan cheese and grating it, leaving many scratches on the underside of the skin. This grating creates a swathe of mini-injuries and, for the next six months, all these carefully placed scratches, as they heal, slowly contract and draw together, tightening the neck. In a way, the doctor starts the ball rolling, but it's the skin itself that does all the real work. Think of an appendix scar, for example, which is much smaller six months after the surgery than it is when first healed. Nature's way of healing tissue includes shrink-ing, and that's the trick of the microsuction—as the months go by, the neck wonderfully tucks up under the chin, while the pa-tient and I watch with great pleasure and joy.

Afterward

Afterward, there is no need for elaborate bandaging, rather an elastic garment is placed under the neck and tied over the top of the head. This garment is a compression device that acts as a sculpturing form to start the shape changes that make this pro-cedure a success. The garment is worn for the first twenty-four hours and then overnight for two weeks more. The patients go home and can bathe, shampoo, and go out the next day. If there is bruising or swelling, it is usually low on the neck where a tie, scarf, or turtleneck sweater will cover it.

Everyone is sent home with three kinds of pills—one for pain (which is seldom needed), one to help with sleep if the excite-ment of the day makes that difficult, and a week's worth of an-tibiotics to minimize the risk of infection.

No matter how often I tell patients at the consultation and just before surgery that the full benefit won't be seen for four to six months, people naturally want the results yesterday. The good news is that real improvement is plainly visible after just a few weeks. Carefully taken office photos prior to surgery help because the patients can then compare their present look with the original pictures to see how far they've come.

The Results

When I began doing microsuction in 1990, I had no idea how long the results would last. I knew it couldn't be permanent be-cause aging never stops and gravity never stops pulling the skin on our necks down. The amazing part is that the vast majority of people I treated at the beginning—no matter how severe the problem, no matter how old the person—have lost no benefit. Seven or eight years later I see these people bringing in friends, or coming in for different procedures, looking as good as when their microsuction was first performed.

Complications

Besides the usual postop concerns of bleeding and infection (both are rare), it is typical for people to feel lumps under the chin (that I call rubbery rocks) for the first few weeks; these are from harmless bleeding under the skin, are not important, and slowly go away. It is pretty typical to have temporary areas of numbness in a patchy distribution of the skin, and even in the lower lip, and this also slowly goes away. Other complications can include asymmetry (although if the same amount of fat is removed from each side, this will rarely happen) and denting or streaking of the skin where the tunnels were made underneath.

The Cost

Neck microsuction can cost from $2,000 to $4,000, depending on the area of the country and the skill and reputation of the person doing the surgery.

FREQUENTLY ASKED QUESTIONS

What about men with heavy turkey necks?

This procedure almost seems to work the best when the problem is the worst. I've had men tell me their necks were so droopy that the oil of the neck skin would consistently stain their ties.

Six months after surgery their necks are much tighter, they look younger, and the substantial savings on dry cleaning bills pays for the surgery in very short order!

Does neck microsuction work on everyone?

No. In the vast majority of people this wonderful technique can replace a lower facelift, but there are some who have thin necks where a classic facelift would be preferred. Many people ask me if there is a way to fix wrinkled skin on the very bottom of the neck. This technique does not correct that area. In fact, there's little that can be done here through any technique; wrinkled neck skin is one of the great unsolved challenges of cosmetic surgery. New erbium lasers, for the first time ever, hold great promise for improving wrinkly lower necks, backs, and hands.

How will I look the next day?

Most people have some bruising and swelling, but the bruising is usually on the very bottom of the neck, where it can be hidden. (Foundation makeup applied over the bruises will conceal them.) This is a good Friday afternoon surgery for people who need to be back at work on Monday.

When can I bathe and work out?

Bathing and even shampooing are fine the next day, and exercising in just a few days. This is a very convenient surgery, and when compared to a lower facelift, it is like a walk in the park.

Chapter 5

GONE TODAY,
HAIR TOMORROW

THE HAIR TRANSPLANT

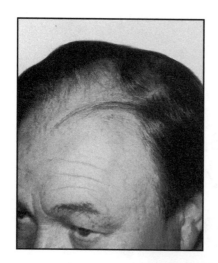
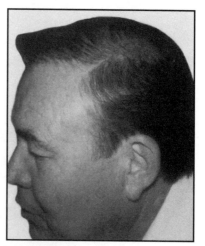
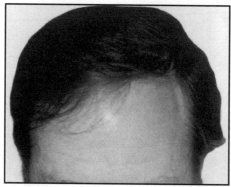
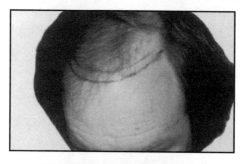

Mini Graph Hair Transplants—before and after

At the ripe age of nineteen I was elected president of the Dartmouth College Class of '67 "Receding Hairline Club." Since my dad had been bald for as long as I could remember, losing my hair wasn't that much of a surprise, but even so, the last thing you want to worry about at your first freshman mixer, beyond the usual acne and social jitters, is whether your date will notice the receding hair at your temples and your thinning crown. So some of us who were worried about hair loss formed the Receding Hairline Club, very much in the way that people in a leaky lifeboat sing songs as they go down to their watery demise. I was president because, every three months, all the members would meet and compare how much hair they'd lost; since I always seemed to have lost the most, I was elected.

Why do I now, at the age of fifty-three, have a decent and totally natural head of hair? With the techniques cosmetic surgeons have at their disposal today, you and the people you love will never have to be president of any club for baldies.

Not Every Inheritance Is a Blessing

There are hundreds of diseases that can cause baldness, but the typical male pattern hair loss (as well as the female variant) is not a disease, but a natural event that is inherited from our parents and arrives with age. All the shampoos that let the hair follicles "breathe," the machines with flashing lights and heat lamps, and the massages that "increase blood flow to the scalp" are all complete consumer frauds when it comes to reversing or even slowing down male-pattern hair loss. This kind of hair loss is natural—but I'm not saying it's desirable or that you should have to live with it.

The exact way we pass on the balding trait to our children is not understood; it's not even known whether the predisposition to baldness is inherited from your father's or your mother's side of the family. The most plausible current explanation is that the trait is dominant, but its expression (the actual amount of hair loss and how early in life it starts) is so complicated that no one can predict what will happen to any individual. You don't, however, need to be a trained geneticist to know that if every male and some of the females in your family have had hair loss, you probably will too. Sometimes, however, this inherited trait can hop and skip over several generations before rearing its head once again.

Just having the trait is not enough; you also have to have the male hormone testosterone; it's the testosterone acting on the genetically susceptible follicles that leads to hair loss. I often tell patients that eunuchs in the court of China never went bald for this reason, and most of them feel this is a little too high a price to pay to remain hirsute. Some, however, claimed that if they'd been offered the choice at a certain point in their lives, it might not have been a difficult decision! If male hormone is the key, why do so many women experience thinning hair as they get older? Unfortunately, in this case, it's normal for women to make just a bit of male hormone, and this little bit is enough to act on those predisposed hairs later in life.

New York City dermatologist Dr. Norman Orentreich is the father of modern hair transplant surgery, and the question he asked himself (and answered) in the 1950s was simple but fundamental. Everyone knew that, even on the baldest man, the fringe of remaining hair above the neck and the ears generally stays for life. Why was that? What made this hair resistant to male hormone, and what would happen if you took this hair and implanted it into the totally bald spot on top? In the trade we call the hair moved from the fringe area the donor hair and the bald skin you move it to the recipient area. Dr. Orentreich was the one who proved that the persistent lifetime fringe hair was donor dominant, meaning that, no matter where you transplant and move this hair—to the bald scalp, the leg, the hand, anywhere—it always remembers its original programming and will live for as long in the new area as it would have in the fringe.

This was great news because it meant you could artfully move hair from the fringe, where there was a surplus, to the bald front and crown. Every person who has had a hair transplant (as well as every person who performs hair transplants) owes Dr. Orentreich a debt of gratitude as the father and pioneer of this technique.

Hair Loss Is Almost Never a Good Thing

Because our hair is such a source of pleasure and pride in our lives, losing it can be a great source of pain and anxiety. For many men, hair loss may feel like a loss of virility, of being less than you once were. For teenagers, it it can be socially paralyzing, since a teen who's nearly bald can look ten or more years older than his actual age, and this makes dating very difficult.

Women can be so creative with hairstyles to hide thinning that few people realize how many are losing their hair, but for some women, the hair can become so thin that no styling or layering will prevent balding scalp from showing through. I have consulted with many women over the years who are simply devastated by the prospect of hair loss. Most balding men and women are willing to try any remedy that might slow down or reverse their hair loss, and this has made hair transplants one of the most popular and enduring of cosmetic surgery procedures. No matter what stage your loss, hair transplants make everyone look younger and feel more confident.

You Gotta Have Art

The technique, however, is no walk in the park, as the hair transplant surgeon must be a combination of artist, technician, and psychologist, and additionally must be able to look far into the future of a patient's life. Most of you come to us as the hair loss is progressing, some sooner than others. The younger the patient and the more recent the balding, the more difficult it is for a doctor to plan the work.

I worry the most when a young male in his late teens or early twenties comes in just as the thinning hair starts to show. At that age, it's almost impossible to know how quickly or extensively the balding may progress. There is so much extra hair on the scalp that you can lose tens of thousands of hairs and not notice anything at all. Additionally, the rate of loss is erratic and unpredictable; sometimes there may be much noticeable thinning when we are very young. The hair loss may then stop for decades, and start again in midlife. Finally, the hair transplanter can only harvest and move so much of the fringe hair (perhaps up to 40 to 50 percent of it over time) to avoid creating gaping bald spots above the collar. You don't want to use up all the available transplantable hair when the patient is young and the full extent of future balding is unknown. The most important thing to remember about a hair transplant is that it doesn't create or add a single hair to your head; it just creatively takes what you have and moves it around to make the most of it.

The problem for the surgeon is that a solution that may work well for a patient in his twenties may end up looking awkward and unnatural later in life. A good rule of thumb for a doctor is to be very, very conservative with young patients. I have noticed that the younger the patient is at the consult, the lower they want me to place the front edge of the hairline, because they can remember very clearly in the recent past how low it was naturally. The problem with this approach is that to duplicate the low hairline of youth misses the fact that even men destined to keep great heads of hair naturally experience some receding as they age.

A telltale unnatural transplant can be seen when forehead wrinkles start appearing in the scalp. When we are young, we have few if any horizontal wrinkles on the forehead, but as we get older, horizontal wrinkles extend up the forehead as the hairline recedes, and if they get too close to the forward edge of a transplant, it gives the game away. The way to stay out of trouble here is to keep the transplanted hairline high enough so that no matter how wrinkled the forehead becomes, and how far the hair eventually thins out, you will have a natural, slightly receded hairline that works at any age.

Another pitfall of starting a hairline too low on a young person is that as the hair loss marches back toward the crown, the doctor could easily run out of donor hairs, leaving the front hairline to fend for itself as an isolated island in a sea of bald skin. I've never run out of donor hairs, but I have sometimes had a patient come back ten years after the initial transplant having lost much more hair than I ever anticipated, and I only had just enough remaining fringe donor hair to extend the transplant. The possibility of running out of donors is one of those things that causes people like me to lose sleep at night. The older the patient and the more complete the hair loss, the easier it is to make a plan that will never let you down later.

None of this means, however, that you can't do great work that looks good for a lifetime on young people with unstable, rapidly receding hairlines, and I'm not suggesting that you wait until you are old and bald before having a transplant. In fact, the only reason that I've never been bald is that I began my transplants the first moment I could, and so can you. It just means that when you go to an expert who specializes in hair transplant surgery, listen to the doctor; you're paying them for their advice and experience. I simply won't take on as a patient anyone who won't listen to me on this issue; I may think of my patients as my employers, but part of being a good employee is not letting the boss convince me to make mistakes in the short run that can have severe consequences later on.

Hair texture, hair color, and skin color are very important in the planning of hair replacement; it's harder to get good coverage when the skin and hair are in contrast. Jet black hair on a very light-skinned scalp is really tough, because no matter how much hair you transplant, you almost always see that scalp shining through. For light-skinned people, blonds do have more fun because the skin and hair are almost the same color and, because there's little contrast, even a little hair looks great.

As the man with dark hair and light skin ages, that distinguished salt-and-pepper look and graying make thin hair in general (as well as hair transplants) look thicker, but the reverse holds true for people with darker skin. For those whose skin and hair are dark, just a small transplant is usually enough when the person is young, but as the hair grays, more hair may need to be transplanted to hide the increasing color contrast between skin and hair color. Here, coloring the hair to hide the gray can help.

Texture is very important. Some hair is thick and some is thin; some is straight and some is curly. It almost goes without saying that if you have gotten this far in the chapter, you already know that thick, full-bodied, curly hair covers more scalp and is easier to work with than thin, straight hair.

A Lesson in the Life of Your Hair

Patients very commonly go to a dermatologist when they suddenly notice a great deal of extra hair shedding. One of the first questions asked is always whether this means the beginning of male-pattern hair loss. The answer is always no. Believe it or not, even for those who are destined to become completely bald, there is no extra hair loss on a daily basis, and losing a lot of hair all at once is usually an indication of some other kind of disease. What happens is that individual hairs, like people, need to take vacations and rest now and then. After years of uninterrupted growth, a single hair will shed and the follicle under the skin will rest and remain dormant for several months, before going back to work to produce a new hair.

We notice these vacationing hairs in the comb or in the shower drain as the normal shedding of about a hundred or more hairs each day. But for every hundred or so shed, about the same number are just back from holiday and beginning to grow again, and there is no net gain or loss. When we are young, the hairs grow for very long periods of time and rest very little; that's why when children's hair is allowed to grow, it can grow to several feet in length. As we get older, however, the growing period shortens in relation to the resting phase, and in male pattern hair loss the growing phase shortens too much. The reason that we go bald, then, is not because we lose extra hair on any given day, but because many of the follicles that go off on vacation never come back to work.

How a Hair Transplant Works

Donor hair can be harvested in a number of ways. After the skin is numbed with local anesthetic (Lidocaine), the original method uses a motorized, rotating cookie cutter to remove small circles of skin and hair about one-sixth of an inch in diameter. Each circle is called a plug and contains about eight to twelve hairs. Remember, this hair is only removed from areas of the fringe just above the collar or ears; the small holes in the back heal all on their own and leave no observable scar. This is the way my first transplant was done and it worked just fine for me.

A newer method is to remove thin strips of skin in the low fringe that extends from ear to ear and to sew the resulting wound closed. The advantage here is that lengths of the strip can be sliced to yield bits of donor material that contain as few or as many hairs as you want, and the surgeon is able to completely customize the work. If you've ever sat at a sushi bar and watched the chef cut, you'll get the idea how this trend has developed, and I call this strip technique the sushi transplant.

The doctor or technicians can mince these long strips into as many as several thousand grafts in a single session, each containing one or two hairs (micrografts), three to four hairs (minigrafts), or even more. Because a hair transplant often requires more than one session, you can go back to the donor area more than once to reharvest.

After the plugs or strips have been readied, the balding skin is then numbed by local anesthetic. If the donors were removed as plugs, slightly smaller holes are made in the recipient scalp and the plugs are gently put in with fine forceps (medical tweezers). The reason for the smaller holes is that skin stretches, and you want the donor hair to have a snug (but not tight) fit in its new home. Hair grafts never need to be sewn or glued into place because, within a few moments, the body fluid in the recipient wound acts as a bond to grip the plug.

If the donor hair has been harvested by the sushi method, the micrografts or minigrafts may be inserted either into a tiny hole in the recipient skin made with a special needle or into a slit made with a medical blade. Here again the body grips the graft. In all cases, space needs to be left between the grafts, just as when a farmer plants seeds, because if the grafts are too close together there will not be enough blood supply to support them and there will not be an optimal amount of hair growth. The smaller the graft size, the closer they can be planted together. Some doctors try to do the whole hair transplant on a bald area in a single session, but in the vast majority of cases, several sessions (separated by a three- to six-month period) are better so that the growth from one visit can start before additional hair is grafted. This will usually achieve the most natural and attractive results.

The needs of every thinning hair patient are so unique that it's a blessing to have the ability to use minigrafts, micrografts, and even small and large plugs, all on the same person. An example of this is the creation of a front hairline. I mentioned earlier that a higher hairline generally looks best because, as you age, it continues to look natural. But how do you actually create that hairline? Here is where the artist comes in.

The next time you go to a forest, notice how the trees are spaced. Every forest (unless it's been completely artificially planted) works the same way: The edge has small trees, spaced widely apart, and as you walk deeper into the woods, the trees get taller, thicker in girth, and more closely spaced. This is exactly the way a doctor should create a hairline, and nothing looks worse than the doll's head, picket fence, pluggy look of a hairline that begins with a bang on the forehead with row after row of tightly packed, fat hair plugs side by side. In the early days, before the advent of minis and micros, it took an unusually gifted surgeon and a patient with just the right combination of skin color, hair color, and texture to avoid this.

As I work on the hairline, I'll walk through the forest, placing the micrografts with one or two hairs liberally spaced in the very front, then using minigrafts with two to four hairs in them and space them more closely together. Several inches behind the front I'll use small plugs to provide the kind of density not possible with mini- and micrografts. I like to use finer, thinner hair in the front and thicker, coarser hair as I move back for added density. In this way, a totally natural hairline can be built up that will fool even your barber.

Just like in real life, doctors and surgical advances are frequently subject to trends. At the big medical meetings a few years back, everyone hailed the death of the old-fashioned hair plug. Any doctor who admitted using full-sized plugs in the back of the hairline to achieve greater density would have been driven out of town on a rail. But when I think about my own hair transplant sessions over the years (I've had three), I am happy I had the minis and micros at the very front for camouflage, and I'm equally happy that in the back I have thick plugs to give me the kind of density I want. In recent journal articles, not surprisingly, the much-vilified plug is making a comeback. After more than twenty years of attending meetings on all kinds of surgical procedures, I sometimes think good ideas from the past are shunned so that the presenter's ideas will look like something dramatically new.

Years ago, one of the saddest consults I could do would be with a man who was so bald that not only was the top totally without hair, but the fringe area was so low and small that no transplant was possible. Remember, you can artfully move up to about half the fringe hair without seeing a thinning, but many people have bald scalps that are larger in surface area than the entire fringe. Even if you moved *all* the fringe hair, which is impossible, it wouldn't cover the top. To start a hair transplant on such a man would be a catastrophe, because you'd run out of donor hair before the work was done and the result would look completely artificial.

Transplanting thousands of micrografts, minigrafts or even

thousands of individual hairs in one or several sessions is more effective. When this hair grows in it will not be thick and dense, but it will give a totally natural, thin coverage that works well and looks good. Remember, many people thin as they age (well, at least their hair does), without going completely bald. This thin growth on top never looks artificial because, when hair is planted singly or in tiny groups, people don't notice the scalp as they would if there were clumps of thick hair growing from plugs and separated by bald skin.

Scalp Reduction and Extension

The scalp is pliable and rubbery, something like a thick, stretched balloon. In the late 1970s, dermatologists developed a technique to cut out large patches of bald scalp on top and on the crown instead of covering these areas with precious, irreplaceable hairs from the fringe. The technique came to be known as scalp reduction, and it rapidly gained popularity because it was a single procedure done under local anesthetic, replaced a technique that normally required hundreds of grafts, and because the benefit could be seen immediately. For men whose donor hair supply would have only been sufficient to transplant the front area, a scalp reduction also made it possible to cover the back because of the dramatically reduced bald spot.

The drawback is that the scar needs to be covered with donor hair. In the early days of the procedure, the scars went right down the middle of the scalp, and, until that scar was covered, not too many of my patients wanted to be sitting down when people around them were standing up, since it looked as though they'd had some strange kind of brain surgery. Subsequently, the scars were either hidden in the fringe itself or the surgeon used what was called the Mercedes procedure (named not from the cost of the surgery but from the fact that the scar is shaped like the Mercedes Benz logo) to further remove bald skin and make the scar less apparent. Another difficulty with this technique was that, several months after the surgery, the scalp would stretch (doctors call it "stretch back") and some (but not all) of the benefit was lost. This stretch back really decreased the popularity of scalp reduction for some doctors (including me), but the technique is still performed by many.

In order to limit stretch back, a technique called scalp extension has recently gained popularity. In this surgery, an elastic device that acts like a rubber band is temporarily placed under the balding scalp and it pulls the fringe slowly together. In a way, this device stretches the scalp prior to scalp reduction so that more bald skin can be removed with less stretch back than when scalp reduction is performed alone.

Follicular Transplants

If you take a simple magnifying glass and look at the scalp, you'll notice that hairs do not grow singly or randomly, but in groups of one to four. Each person has his or her own unique grouping and, in follicular transplants, the idea is to move the hairs as follicular units to more closely mimic the natural growth and patterning. Thousands of these units can be moved in a single session, and some men can be finished in one procedure. This new idea is being embraced by more and more surgeons, and only time will tell if the method yields natural results.

The Preparation

The blood supply to the scalp, particularly in the donor area above the collar, is very large. The usual rules about not having aspirin or aspirin-containing products for two weeks before surgery and no alcohol for at least a week before are even more important than usual. Alcohol and aspirin greatly increase bleeding, and I have been in situations where bleeding was so excessive I almost had to stop the surgery. When I work on one of my regular patients, I can always tell if they've had an aspirin or a beer just before the surgery because it makes their usual bleeding much worse—and I don't appreciate it at all. All patients are also required to have a blood test that screens them for anemia or a hidden bleeding tendency.

At the end of a hair transplant, the scalp is bandaged with a wrap that is a miracle of architecture. Teflon pads, heavily greased with antibiotic ointment, lay directly over the donor area and the grafts, so that when you remove the bandage one or two days later, all the transplanted hairs don't come off with it. On top of the Teflon pads are layers of gauze to absorb any drainage, topped by layers of Ace bandages to keep the whole affair from flying apart. Putting on this contraption takes twenty minutes and requires the nurse to have engineering and artistic skills without parallel. The finished turban is nearly as wide as your shoulders, and we have to tell patients to come in with shirts that button, because it is impossible to slip a pullover shirt over the head wrap. Would it surprise you to know that the vast majority of first-time (and even repeat) patients come in with pullover tops?

Unless you've had it happen to you, this will only be of theoretical interest. On one of my own hair transplants I did everything wrong as a patient. The next morning I took off my bandage without any assistance from my wife, and, much to my horror, about fifteen grafts stuck to the bandage and went down the shower drain. Thank goodness this has never happened to one of my patients.

The Procedure

Hair transplants and scalp reductions are outpatient surgeries done under local anesthesia only or with local anesthesia and IV (intravenous) sedation. I usually numb the donor fringe area first and then the bald scalp. The donor hair is taken, usually by removing narrow strips of skin with the attached hair. Then the sushi chefs (my assistants) take over and cut the hair into various sizes from singles hairs to bits of skin containing two, three, four, or more hairs. Then the slits are cut in the bald scalp.

Especially when creating a natural front hairline, it is great to have grafts of every size spread out before me like the colors of an artist's palette. As described before, single hairs of fine texture, widely spaced apart, go in the very front. Then as I work from front to back I use larger and larger grafts of coarser texture to increase density. This whole process can take up to six to eight hours when moving thousands of minis and micros at one sitting.

Scalp reductions take less than an hour. I draw a circle with a marker all around the head at a level just above the ears. I go around the head injecting local anesthetic until the whole top is numb. This takes less than ten minutes, and I always know the patient is ready when he tells me he feels like he's wearing a hat that's three sizes too small. After a scalp reduction there is no bandage, the scalp is cleaned, and the patient goes home without any visible sign of having had surgery.

Afterward

After carefully removing the transplant turban the next day, patients shower and can even shampoo their hair, but very carefully, in a way so as not to dislodge the grafts. If the patient is totally bald on top, there will be small scabs where the donor grafts were placed in the recipient skin for up to two weeks. It helps if you have the type of job where keeping a hat on doesn't attract attention. For people who are just filling in thin areas where there is still plenty of hair, the scabs usually don't show.

I tell patients not to engage in strenuous work or exercise because the increased blood pressure could cause bleeding around the hair, which could in turn dislodge the grafts. Men, being men, often ask me if they can engage in amorous activities, and I say yes if they are not too active (if I said no, would they really listen?). I always imagine that if a man were to raise his blood pressure enough the plugs would pop out like champagne corks. This has never happened, but theoretically it could. Stitches in the donor area, if present, come out in two weeks. There is very little pain after a hair transplant, but sometimes there is a headache the day after a scalp reduction from the stretching of the skin.

The Results

About two weeks after a hair transplant, the vast majority of the transplanted hair falls out by the roots. I always tell this to my patients at the consultation because it would really worry anyone who had not been forewarned. For the short time the hair is out of the body, between being harvested and then replaced in its new home, it has no direct blood supply. This is a real shock to the follicle and causes the shedding of the transplanted hair.

I often compare this to transplanting a flowering plant from one part of the garden to another. If it was in bloom, all the flowers will usually fall off because the plant is struggling to put roots into the soil. The exact same thing is true for your transplanted hair, but there's no need to worry; the follicle you need to host the transplanted hair is intact and healthy for the rest of your life.

For the first six weeks, the follicle is getting itself acclimatized to its new home and is not much worried about making a hair. The new hairs begin to grow two to three months later. Once started, you can't stop them, and they will grow at the same speed and texture they previously did. For a first-time patient, feeling the stubble as the hairs just come through the skin is a great experience. Once this happens, patients know the surgery has worked, but they still don't know if the transplant will give them the coverage they want because the hair is still too short.

For most of us, hair grows on average about one inch a month. This means that until the hair reaches a length of two or more inches in men or longer in women, you can't style it. Only when the transplanted hairs reach the length you like will the full impact of the surgery be apparent and only then will you know how well it worked.

This whole process, from the day of surgery to hair you can style and work with, takes six to nine months. That's why I tell patients to go slowly and not schedule sessions too closely together. Before the days of minigrafts, when only large plugs were used, there was good reason to do sessions as quickly as you could, because a single session looked really obvious as the clumps of hair grew in. In those days, sometimes I'd do three sessions in the first six months to get adequate coverage to hide the tufted look of large plugs. Transplants with minis and micros look completely natural, even in totally bald men, after a single session. One session may not give you the density you want, but patience really pays off when undergoing a hair transplant because, after seeing the full impact of a session, you and your doctor will be better able to plan for the future.

Complications

Infections can occur after hair transplant or scalp reduction, but are very rare, though I routinely put people on a course of antibiotics just to be sure. I've rarely seen postoperative bleeding from the donor site, but this could be stopped with firm hand pressure over the wound or by placing a stitch over the bleeding area. Once in a great while there is tremendous swelling over the front part of the scalp and forehead that begins two to three days after the transplant, lasts four or five days, and then subsides on its own. This does no harm to the hairs, but can be very alarming to the patient, and can be so great in the forehead and down to the middle face as to make the patient look like half-man, half-ape missing link.

One of the key technical skills the surgeon needs is to watch the direction of the hair as it leaves the scalp from the donor fringe. Hair has a direction, bias, and nap, like fabric. It's important in a hair transplant that, as the donor fringe is minced into the grafts of all different sizes, the cut be perfectly parallel with the living part of the follicle. If the cut is at a tangent, the living follicle at the base of the hair will be injured and will never put out a growing hair again. But no matter the skill of the surgeon, not every transplanted hair will grow.

The Cost

Scalp reductions cost from $1,500 to $3,000 or more, since very often people need more than one to reduce a large bald spot. Micrografts and minigrafts cost from $4 to $10 for each graft, but remember, some doctors transplant a thousand of these per session. You can safely bet that for a very bald man, the total expense can easily be $10,000 to $20,000 over time. If you consider the labor involved and the skill needed to do a good job, you can see that this cost is reasonable, and the results, after all, will be with you your entire life.

More people than not come in as their hair is just beginning to thin. For them a single session might do, and another session might not be needed for many years, when the nontransplanted hair has also thinned. In this case, the patient will probably spend about the same amount as the already bald man who does it all at once, but the expense is spaced out over time.

FREQUENTLY ASKED QUESTIONS

Can I get a haircut on the transplanted hair?

Yes. Getting haircuts again is one of the great joys after a hair transplant. Your hairstylist will have to work harder than in the past to cut this newly flourishing hair. Hair from the fringe is young at heart and will grow very long after it's transplanted, if you want it to. It will also grow with its original texture and color; if it was curly, it will stay that way, and if it came from graying temples, it will color that way as well. Though a hair transplant generally makes all people look much younger, this can be an exception.

You can style, color, curl, or even hang by this hair. It is your hair. Don't baby it. Treat it the way you would have if you'd never had hair loss.

Rogaine: Does it work?

Rogaine is a product that has FDA approval as a treatment for hair loss; my experience is that it has very limited usefulness. In fact, for a truly bald scalp where no hair has grown for years, I've never seen it do anything. After long-term use, it can grow a small amount on about one-third of those with male pattern hair loss, with results that are more like peach fuzz than typical thick hair. It stimulates the hair follicles in a way that no one really understands yet, and it needs to be applied to the scalp twice a day. All the extra hair growth that it stimulates will be lost as soon as you stop using it. The expense and inconvenience of using this lotion twice a day for life to grow a few hairs seems a waste to me. Rogaine is, however, useful for slowing hair loss, and I recommend it for this purpose.

**Is it true that there are now pills that can regrow
hair in balding men?**

Last month the FDA approved for the first time ever the use
of the chemical Finasteride (brand name is Propecia by Merck
and Co., Inc.) in pill form for regrowing hair in balding men.
The FDA approved Finasteride in 1994 to treat benign enlargement of the prostate gland in men. It was noted that many of the
men who took this pill to shrink their enlarged prostate saw a
visible increase in hair in their scalps.

Propecia works by blocking an essential enzyme responsible
for male pattern hair loss. Increased numbers of hairs can be
seen as soon as three months after taking the pill and this increases over the next year. Though the hair growth occurs more
in the crown than the front of the scalp, the regrowth is significant. Finasteride also has been proven to slow down or even
halt hair loss. Side effects were uncommon, with less than 2 percent of men having a decreased libido. This product is very un-
likely to make hair thick and bushy, but it is a great advance.

Chapter 6

FILLING WRINKLES

THE FAT REINJECTION TECHNIQUE

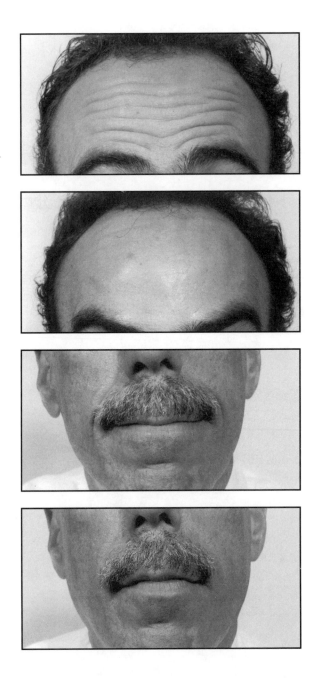

(above) Eliminating wrinkles with Botox—before and after
(below) Laughlines filled with Softform—before and after

A newborn baby has virtually no lines on its face, and it's a marvel of life that, as we leave our teenage years and enter our twenties and thirties, we develop the kind of expressive lines around the eyes and mouth that add character and uniqueness to our appearance. But as the years go by, these become the deep lines of advancing age, and our best friends ask us if we're tired after a good night's rest or if we're angry about something, even if we've just won the lottery. At some point, a lifetime of expression, laughter, and sun imprints the kind of deep lines on the face that are no fun to look at in the bathroom mirror and that may inspire you to call someone like me.

In this chapter we will go over how cosmetic surgery can improve the deep lines around the mouth and forehead, and even plump up the lips, while the next chapter, "Skin Resurfacing," will tell you how to improve fines lines such as crow's feet, lipstick lines, and cheek lines. Best of all, reread chapter 2 for the latest information on how to slow down the onset of wrinkles and use nonprescription creams and lotions to soften the ones you already have.

Collagen

Collagen is the supporting connective tissue that gives the skin its strength. We never notice collagen until we begin to lose it, a sign of which is deepening wrinkles on the face. The logic of replacing the collagen to improve wrinkles was not a great leap of imagination on the part of scientists; the main problem was where to find donors. I've met very few people who want to donate their own skin to friends and neighbors to help them look younger, but happily there's a relatively simple solution. People and animals have regularly been trading tissue for many years, with insulin and heart valve replacements being the obvious examples. In the case of collagen, the best donor animals are cows. In fact, several million Americans have had cow collagen injected into the lines of their faces.

The procedure is very simple. At the first visit, the doctor will ask general questions about your health and make sure that you are a good candidate. Just to be sure that you're not allergic, a small amount of collagen is injected under the skin of the forearm and left there for a month. Any unusual redness or swelling could mean that you have allergies to collagen and should either repeat this patch test for confirmation or skip using collagen in your face.

If there's no allergic reaction, you can begin a course of visits that, to put it mildly, will not be much fun. Each individual crow's foot, vertical lip line, and laugh line around the mouth is injected in a manner not very different from the way a sewing needle moves across fabric, with multiple punctures of the skin into which the doctor injects a small amount of the collagen. At the end of the treatment, if you feel the lines with your finger, you will feel small bumps of material, but these bumps soon smooth out, leading to the softening of the wrinkles.

Why would any sane person pay hundreds of dollars per visit to do this? The reason is that experienced physicians can place the collagen quickly, small needles make the pinpricks tolerable, and the convenience of leaving the office fifteen minutes later and going about your normal activities are hard to beat.

In my experience the problem with collagen is that, for most people, it just doesn't last. I have seen very few of my patients keep the results beyond twelve months, and there are so few of these people that I can remember their names. For the majority, in two to six months, the collagen is absorbed as if they'd never had it.

When I first realized this, I called a number of physician friends around the country and felt somewhat reassured when they told me they were having the same problem. To maintain collagen's benefits, you need to visit the doctor at least four times a year, and the repeated expense and inconvenience exhaust even the most diehard patients. I had the embarrassing experience of a patient once telling me that the collagen had completely vanished by the time the patient had gotten the bank statement showing the check made out to me for the visit. When, in 1990, I met Dr. Luiz Toledo in Brazil and learned the fat reinjection technique, that was the end of collagen for me and my patients.

Complications from collagen injections are rare, but can include allergy, infection, swelling, and bruising at the injection site. In the more than ten years that I administered collagen, none of my patients had a serious, long lasting, or harmful complication.

Collagen treatments are charged by the vial (one-thirtieth of an ounce) of collagen, which run $300 to $400 each. A single visit may require the use of more than one vial, and many people need to be retreated every two to three months.

Liquid Silicone

The use of liquid silicone injections to improve lines on the face has been banned by the FDA because, in a number of patients,

the body reacted against this foreign material, causing permanent, visible lumps under the skin. Additionally there've been reports of the silicone migrating to other parts of the body.

I have never understood any physician using or defending the
use of silicone for soft tissue replacement, such as improving facial lines. No matter how skillful the doctor is, in some people
the body will try to reject the silicone and will wall it off, pro-
ducing the characteristic lumps that I see when people who have
gotten the injections from other doctors come to my office.
There is no practical way to remove these lumps except to cut
them out, leaving highly visible scars.

Several years ago, I debated a well-meaning doctor and one
of his patients about this practice on the *Larry King Live* television
show. The patient was an articulate, beautiful woman in her
fifties, and the doctor was proud to say that he had injected silicone into her face for years and that this technique was no
small part of her current beauty. In a way, the doctor was right.
Without the silicone this woman would have looked older. But
no matter how hard I tried, I could convince neither of them
that every visit to get more silicone was like Russian roulette,
the result of which could easily be the destruction of her face.

This doctor also was arguing that the silicone he used was
"medical grade," meaning that it was somehow better than the industrial chemical that came out of vats for industrial use. This
made no sense to me, and it makes no difference to your welfare.
If a doctor is injecting silicone into your face, at best this doctor
is dead wrong, and at worst he or she may be a quick-buck artist
who isn't going to hold your hand when it goes wrong.

Recently, a woman called the office inquiring about the fat
transfer technique for improving her deep facial lines and told
the receptionist that she had been given collagen shots in the
past that had left small, permanent bumps under the skin. I knew
none of the details of her conversation with the front office, but
the moment I walked in for the consultation I knew she had

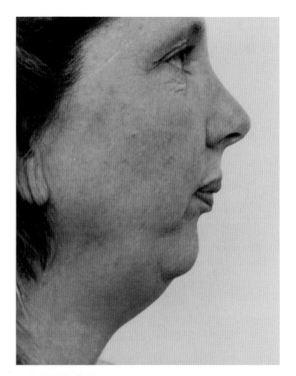
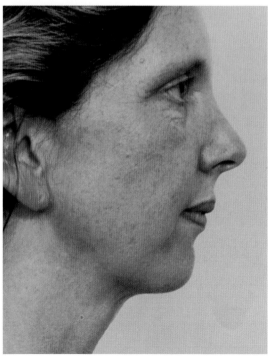

Neck Microsuction—before and after

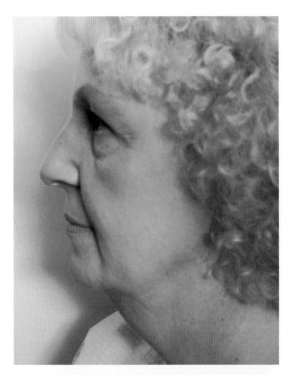

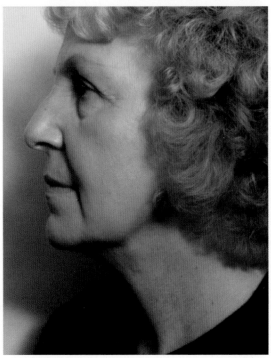

Neck Microsuction—before and after

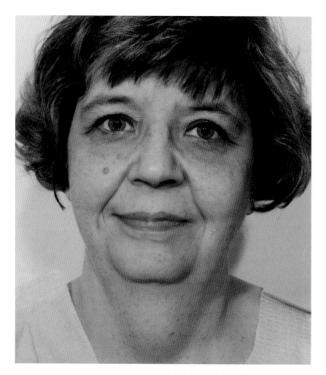

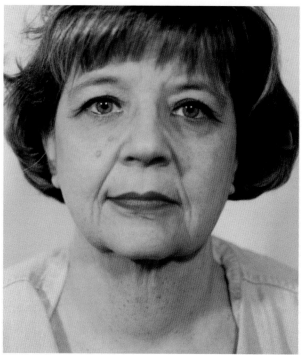

Neck Microsuction—before and after

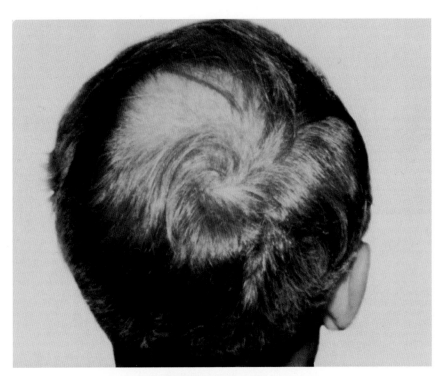

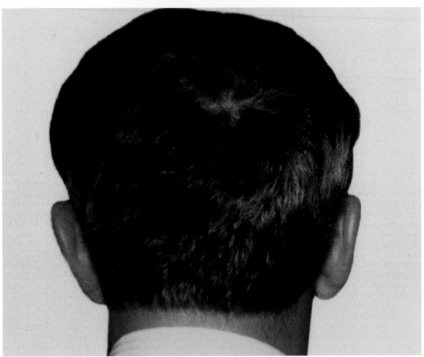

Hair Transplant of the Crown—before and after

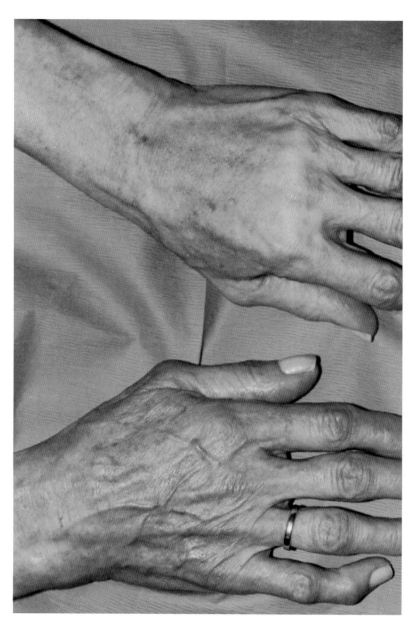

Fat transfer in hands—before and after

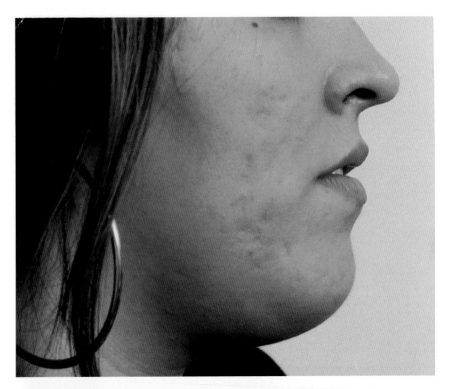
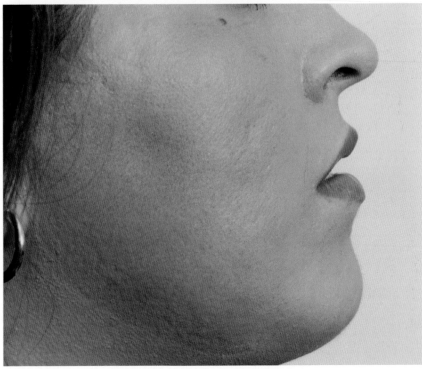

CO2 Laser Skin Resurfacing—before and after

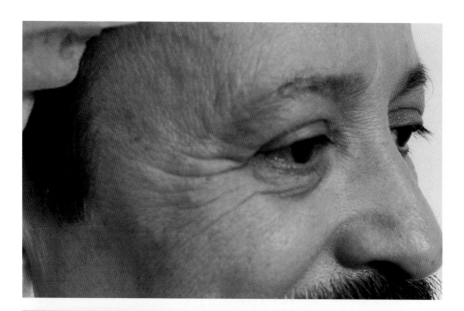

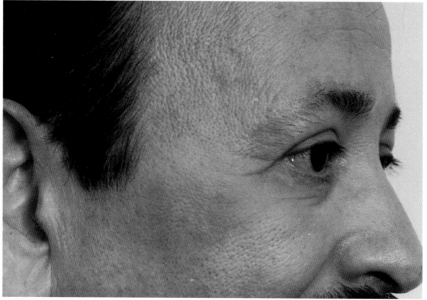

CO2 Laser Skin Resurfacing—before and after

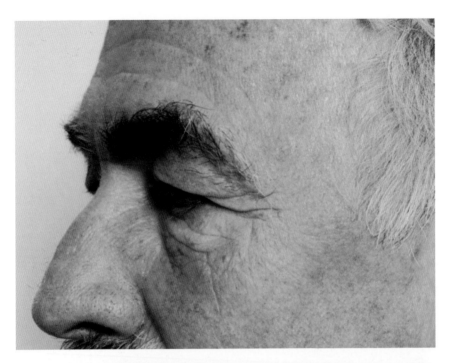

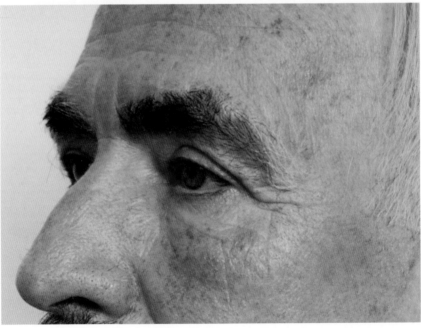

CO2 Laser Upper and Lower Eyelid Lift—
before and after

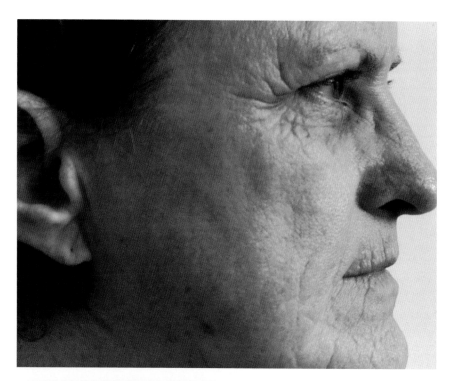
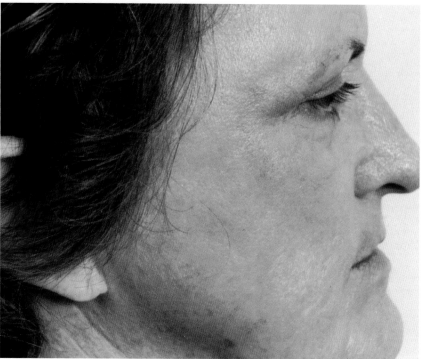

CO2 Laser Skin Resurfacing of eyes and mouth
and CO2 Laser Eyelid Lift —before and after

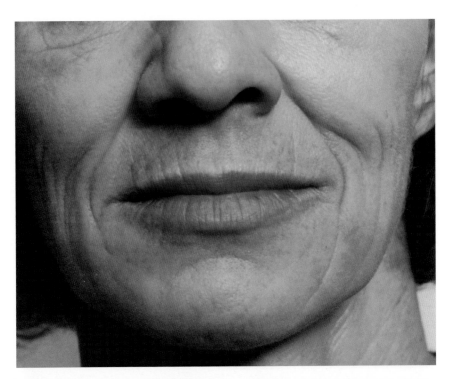

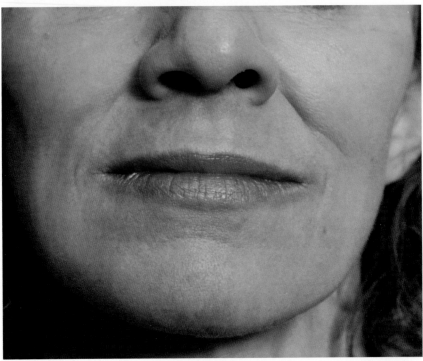

Full facial CO2 Laser Skin Resurfacing, Alternative
Face Lift, and Fat Injections—before and after

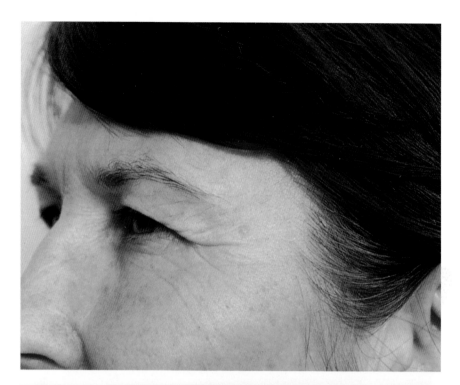
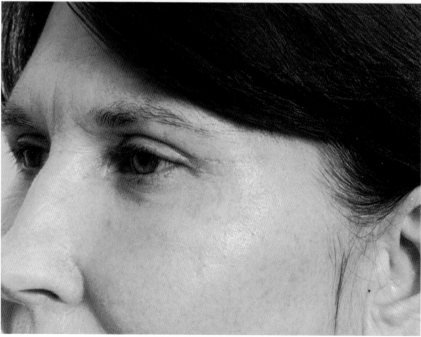

Alternative Face Lift, CO2 Laser Upper and Lower Eyelid Lift, and CO2 Laser Skin Resurfacing of Crow's Feet—before and after

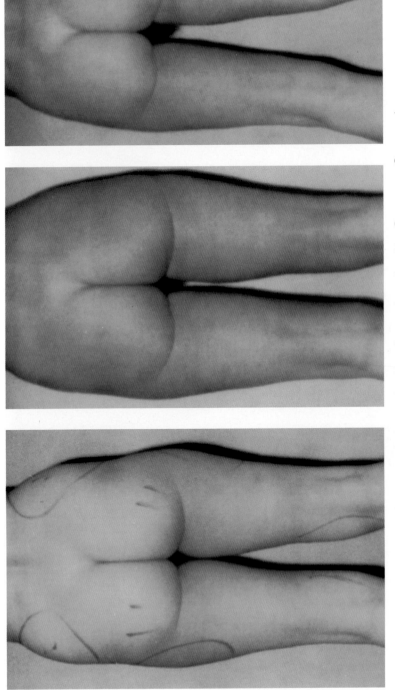

Liposculpture, buttocks raised with Gaynor Cannula (a 55-year old woman!)—before, during, after

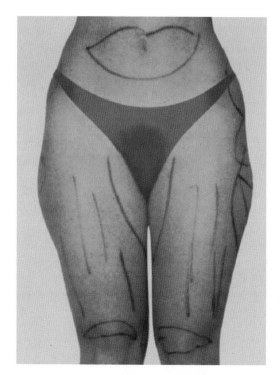

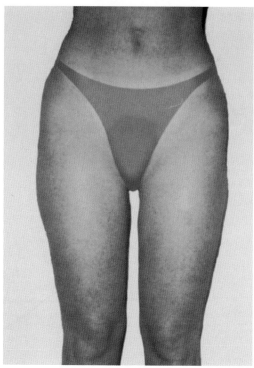

Liposculpture of knees, inner thighs, saddlebags,
and stomach—before and after

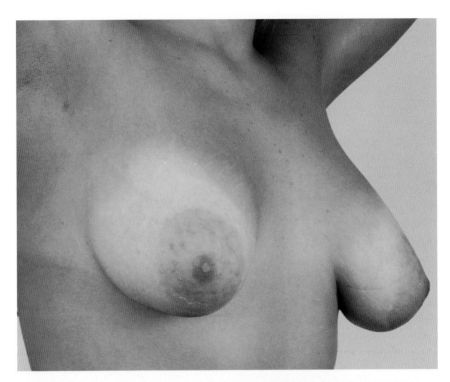

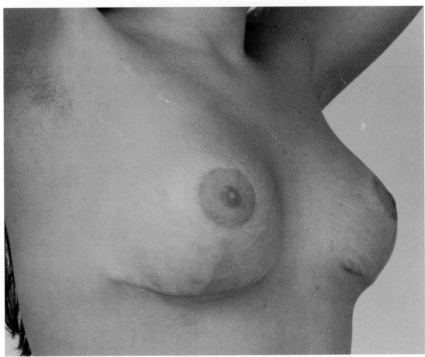

Mastopexy with the inverted T-incision—
before and one year after

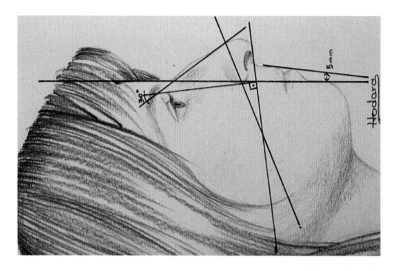

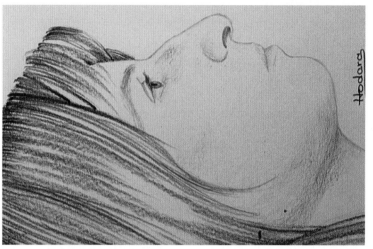

Hodara

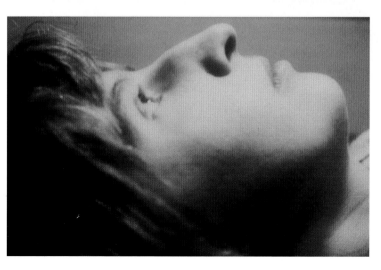

Hodara

Rhinoplasty—before

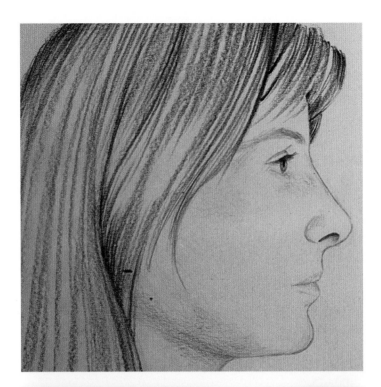
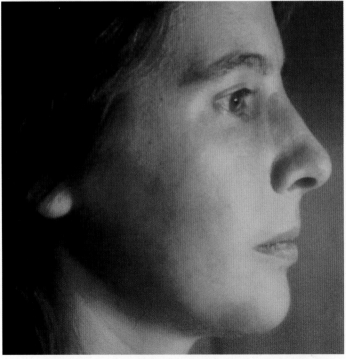

Rhinoplasty—after

been given silicone shots to the face. The lumps silicone leaves under the skin are very characteristic in appearance, and I have seen people with these lumps many times over the years. Over the years I've seen other patients who were told by their doctors they had been given collagen who I am certain were given silicone without their knowledge or permission. Years ago, two of my close, highly skilled physician friends became so frustrated with the short-term benefits of collagen that they began injecting silicone to try to cut down on the need for repetitive, expensive visits to maintain the collagen's effect. Both had patients who developed the typical silicone lumps in a short period of time, and they never used it again.

I've never been accused of being subtle, but I want to make the point with a sledgehammer that liquid silicone injections of the face are unpredictable and dangerous.

Botox

Botox is the trade name for the chemical botulinum toxin, produced by bacteria. It is not a wrinkle filler per se, but instead blocks nerve impulses to muscles. Though it does not sound logical to inject nerve toxins produced by bacteria under the skin, Botox is a very useful treatment. It works best on the deep vertical lines of the forehead between the eyebrows, those wrinkles that make us look angry all the time. These deep furrows are produced by small postage stamp–sized muscles between the eyebrows, and in some people these muscles are so highly developed as a family trait that these deep wrinkles appear early in their teenage years.

After the Botox is injected, nerve impulses to the muscles causing the wrinkles are blocked, the skin magically smooths out, and the wrinkles vanish. The benefit slowly kicks in over a five- to twelve-day period after a simple, short office visit. The drawback is that the results are temporary and in most people will last about six months. Botox visits typically cost $500 to $750 each.

Gortex

When I first heard that doctors were putting Gortex into the face to soften wrinkles and outline the lips, I thought to myself, Isn't that the name of the fabric used in ski clothing to keep us warm? The answer is yes. That wonderful fabric that keeps us from getting frostbitten on ski slopes can be very useful in improving our appearance as well. In medicine, Gortex had been used for many years as suture material in general surgery, and one of its prime medical uses was for sewing deep inside the body, where the suture thread would have to be left for life.

In a brief outpatient procedure done under local anesthetic, Gortex is threaded under the skin of the lips to outline the border between the pink lip skin (the vermillion) and the normal skin. Multiple strands of the thread can be put under the laugh lines around the mouth or the vertical lines of the forehead.

When in Brazil to visit a physician friend, I met a woman who spoke fluent English and who had had an interesting experience with Gortex. She had always wanted a better outline around her lips and so had had the Gortex threaded under the skin, but a few days later she was finishing a meal and a small amount of the thread extruded out of her lip. To solve the problem she took her manicuring scissors out of her purse and clipped off the visible thread. This happened whenever she ate a meal over the next several days, and she finally had to return to the clinic. My doctor friend then pulled the rest of the Gortex out, causing the woman no pain, and replaced it under local anesthesia. Years later the Gortex was still there and the woman was happy to have it.

Other than rare infections or extrusion, Gortex has worked

well for many people, and patients I have met in my practice who have had it are pleased with the results. The cost ranges from $500 to $2000.

Fat Reinjection

The perfect modeling material for filling deep wrinkles would be readily available, perfectly natural, would last long enough to be worth the effort and expense, would involve a relatively short and simple office visit, and would have a cost that matched the value of how much it improved the appearance. Medical science has searched for decades for this perfect material and, low and behold, it was not just under our noses, but under our skin.

That material was the easily available fat in the skin, something every person has plenty of. Over the years, when I have explained to patients the idea of removing it from, say, their hips or chubby knees and transplanting it to the face, their enthusiasm for improving their wrinkles was more than matched by the wonderful idea of taking fat off unwanted areas. Our fat is very useful for plumping up thinning lips as we age, and it works very well to enhance or enlarge cheeks and chins; you can even use it in the backs of the hands to hide veins and fill out the hollow look that develops in all of us as we age. How many woman comedians have used the line that the hands always give away age? Now that is no longer true. It seems like a gift direct from Mother Nature herself that you can now look better by transplanting some of you to you.

The patient usually gets to pick which body area they want to donate the fat from, and this always makes people smile very broadly as they pick from the knees, hips, saddlebags, stomach, and love handles, just to name some of the most popular choices. The chosen area is numbed using a dilute solution of local anesthetic (Lidocaine). After a twenty-minute wait, to be sure that the fat is completely numbed, it's harvested through a small pinhole in the skin using a hollow, blunt instrument called a cannula attached to a small syringe supplying the vacuum needed to extract (but not harm) the fat. Most times I remove about 10 ccs—one-third of an ounce—which is plenty to inject all the lines of the face, cheeks, chin, and lips on a single visit; hands usually get an additional 10 ccs each.

The skin over the wrinkles is numbed using lidocaine, and the fat is injected in long thin lines under the skin so as to build up the indentation. It is very important that the doctor not inject too much fat in any one visit since less of it will last. Just like with hair transplants, if you inject too much at once, the blood supply may not be able to nourish the tissue, and less of the graft will "take."

That's why, in this technique, it's best to do three visits spread over six months. At each visit, the wrinkle or problem area gets a thin layer of fat, time is allowed for the fat to "take," and then an additional layer is added. I charge a single set fee of $750 per visit no matter how many areas are to be done, and I never limit how much fat I harvest.

Over the first six weeks after a visit, not all the fat survives, and in fact more is (harmlessly) absorbed (on average 70 percent) than lives (about 30 percent). This sounds like a great loss, but in comparison to other techniques, fat transfer is very successful. There is no exact medical answer as to why so much is absorbed, but in speaking to many other doctors who have excellent ways to inject fat, the results are roughly similar. Everyone knows how stubborn fat is to get rid of when we eat too much on holidays, but the same stuff becomes very finicky when you try to move it from one home to another. In rare instances, all the fat from the transfer is absorbed and there is a complete loss.

For the vast majority of patients, the fat that does take and survive will stay for many years. One good thing about this high absorption is that the patient's face changes only a little each time, allowing the patient to guide the doctor at each visit to the desired end result.

At the end of a fat transfer visit, the face is somewhat swollen, only rarely bruised, and in general looks presentable in public by the next day. Additionally, there's a slight chance of infection when using this technique.

SoftForm

The absolutely newest idea in battling wrinkles is SoftForm, a permanent implant made from material that's been safely used in more than 3 million vascular surgery patients for the past twenty years. It comes as a soft, round, spongy tube with a hollow center; the length of the tube is trimmed to match the length of the region being treated, and it works terrifically to soften deep wrinkles, such as the laugh lines around the mouth and the deep puppet lines that reach from the corner of the mouth to the chin. Because I personally have always had deep laugh lines, I decided to give SoftForm a try.

An associate in my clinic numbed the nerve that supplies sensation to the area around the mouth and used a little local Lidocaine to numb the laugh lines themselves. (On a scale of from one to ten, with one being no discomfort, the discomfort of this numbing was a two or three). He then made small incisions in the skin at the bottom and top of the laugh lines right in the wrinkles. When he inserted the SoftForm, I felt a bit of pressure, but no real discomfort or pain. He then closed the small openings in the skin with one stitch each (which came out in three days); the whole thing took about twenty minutes.

I had some swelling for three or four days, but no bruising, and the area was slightly tender. I showered the next morning, went to work, and was surprised that no one noticed the small stitches.

The difference it made in the appearance of my laugh lines was amazing to me. What is remarkable about SoftForm is that full-blown facelifts, as you'll learn in chapter 9, do almost nothing for these lines in the central part of the face. I've included before-and-after photographs of my implants so you can see the results for yourself.

The cost is $1,000 to $2,000, depending on how much work is done.

FREQUENTLY ASKED QUESTIONS

How do I get rid of the permanent lumps I feel under the skin from liquid silicone?

There is currently no way to get rid of these lumps, which are often plainly visible, except by surgically cutting the lumps out, leaving an unsightly scar. That is the problem with liquid silicone, and most people live with the lumps of silicone in their faces for the rest of their lives.

How often can I get collagen treatments?

You can get collagen shots as often as two weeks apart. Because collagen is not permanent, it's a good idea to pace yourself so that you don't get it so often that the expense makes you quit altogether. Many of my collagen patients either come in several times a year or come in for a touchup just before a special event, such as a vacation, a wedding, or a new job.

How permanent are fat transfers?

No one knows for sure, but I'm encouraged because every week I see patients who had fat injected as long as eight years ago and the original pictures show that plenty of the fat is still present, improving their looks.

If fat is so long lasting for most people, how come some people come in to do touchups?

No technique to soften wrinkles stops or even slows down the process of aging. After a period of time many patients return for a single touchup visit to work on the new wrinkles that inevitably occur. The process of aging has to do with how much unprotected sun exposure a person gets and with their genetic inheritance. If your parents looked old before their time, you probably will, too.

Chapter 7

SKIN RESURFACING

PEEL, DERMABRASION, AND THE CARBON DIOXIDE LASER

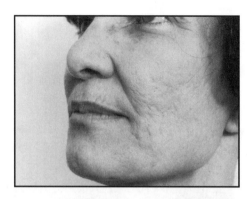

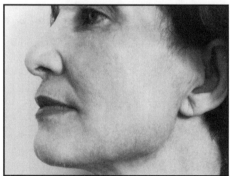

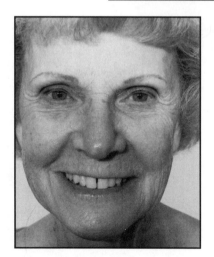 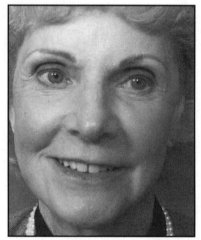

CO_2 Laser Skin Resurfacings—before and after

120

Whatever happened to the perfectly smooth, soft as velvet, all one color, no visible pores skin of our baby pictures? Just about all of us have incredible skin when we're born, but sadly it's all downhill from there. No wonder the creams and lotions that promise to remove our wrinkles and smooth our rough spots are such an enormously popular (and lucrative) business. Every time you turn around there's a new one made of some ingredient no one ever thought of before: turtle oil, avocados, even placentas.

The problem is that nonprescription, over-the-counter creams, by their very nature, have little if any long-term effect on your skin's wrinkles or smoothness. The very fact that you can buy these without a prescription tells you they are almost useless, since our government (in the form of the FDA) would never allow a deeply penetrating cream to be available over the counter. Remember, if some new "miracle" skin product sounds too good to be true, it almost always is just that.

The trained cosmetic surgeon, however, now has methods to

resurface and retexture imperfections in the skin, methods that improve wrinkles and can greatly help scars from acne, chicken pox, traumatic injury, and even scars from cosmetic surgery (though that of course *never* happens). The traditional methods of face peel and dermabrasion are still in use today, though in recent years they've been eclipsed by high-tech lasers. If this book had been written just four or five years ago, I'd have had to spend much more time telling you about various peels and dermabrasion techniques, but now I'll give them only a quick run-through because I feel very strongly that their day has come and gone, except in very rare instances. Though there are many doctors who achieve great results with these older methods and I myself did peels and dermabrasions for many, many years, using them in the wake of what's available now makes little sense. The lasers are so much better it's not even a contest. My state-of-the-art laser setup cost more than $100,000, and I think it has revolutionized my work so much that it's worth every penny.

Dermabrasion

Dermabrasion uses a small, rapidly rotating wheel (fraise) to smooth the skin, and it operates in exactly the same fashion as a sanding machine smoothing wood. This wheel looks very much like a jeweler's grindstone, and in fact the ones I used were studded with industrial diamonds and were very rough to the touch. Because diamonds are the hardest material in all of nature and skin is among the softest, the fraise always wins. Dermabrasion can be very useful to lessen scarring, smooth certain types of wrinkles, and was used in the past to remove tattoos on the lower body. The abrasion of the procedure literally grinds away the top layer of skin, and after healing, a whole new layer is created.

A dermatologist sees skin as varying widely in texture and thickness, depending on where it's located. There's thick, armadillo-like skin on the upper back that's completely different in its anatomy and healing ability from the soft, thin skin of the eyelids. What this means is that the same surgical method that will wonderfully improve acne scars on the face may be disastrous when used to try to improve acne scars on the upper back. Because the skin on areas like the upper back, the legs, upper arms, and stomach is thick, almost all the techniques useful for improving facial wrinkles and scars are unsuitable (and even dangerous) elsewhere. When dermabrasion is tried in these forbidden areas, healing is so erratic and the chance of developing severe, thickened scars so common that I always tell patients I won't even think of it. That is why there are currently no good methods to improve deep wrinkles on the lower neck or severe cystic acne scars on the back.

At the beginning of a dermabrasion, the skin is cleansed with antiseptic and then degreased with rubbing alcohol or acetone (which you may know as nail polish remover). The degreasing is very important because any surface oil can make the penetration inconsistent. Anesthesia can be a combination of IV sedation, regional blocks of the nerves that supply sensation to the face, or even general anesthesia. The deep wrinkles and deep scars are marked beforehand with a special surgical pen, and the doctor uses the depth of penetration of the ink as a guide to how deep they are going on the wrinkle or scar as the pen marks disappear from view.

Just before the fraise is applied, a refrigerant (exactly like the chemical in your refrigerator) is sprayed on the skin to make it numb and stiff. The refrigerant application is a small art in and of itself since the color-making cells of the skin can freeze to death very easily. In this way, small areas are frozen and planed, one after another, in a methodical manner until a larger area (or the whole face) has been treated. This wheel is rapidly rotating hundreds of times per second, and so you want your doctor to have a steady hand and not be a dawdler or daydreamer. The hand movement of the surgeon consists of a series of scalloped arcs, so that at the end there are no streaks or permanent brush marks left as scars on the skin.

As the procedure goes along it gets harder and harder for the surgeon to actually see what he or she is doing because the skin layer is rich with blood vessels. The total amount of blood loss is not harmful, but it drives doctors like me nuts because it gets in the way of fully visualizing what we're doing. Additionally, this blood gets into the air, and even with the best surgical masks, the staff is probably breathing in some of your blood. In this time of frightening blood-borne diseases, such as HIV and hepatitis, the office staff is genuinely at risk.

After the skin has been sufficiently abraded, it is protected with either a layer of antibiotic ointment or one of several specialized bandages that aid in healing. People return the next day for a checkup and then several times per week to make sure all is well. The skin is really red for the first weeks, but it slowly tones down to look like a severe sunburn after two to three weeks, and pancake makeup can usually be applied at that time. Total healing is around two to three months; back to work with camouflage makeup at around two weeks. The downtime from work for a deep dermabrasion, deep peel, or even a deep laser skin resurfacing is about two weeks.

Even in its heyday, dermabrasion was not for everyone. People with darker, olive-colored skin were bad candidates for a dermabrasion since their skin could heal permanently lighter or darker as a result of the technique.

Face Peels

A face peel is the ultimate uncontrolled cosmetic surgery because it depends far more on the art of cosmetic surgery than on the science of medicine. Though the type and strength of the acid used is based on a technique of a kind, it is the experience of the doctor that is everything. Face peels are done with a medical device that can be bought at any discount drugstore or supermarket in America—the venerable Q-tip. For me, deep peels are a thing of the past in favor of the carbon dioxide laser, but many superb doctors do peels today and achieve results that are incredible.

PHENOL PEELS

Phenol is an acid that coagulates (or gels) the tissue of the skin, creating an immediate white frosting, and experienced doctors can tell by the intensity of the whiteness how deep the acid is penetrating. The goal is to penetrate through the outer layer (the epidermis) of the skin and into the top part of the second layer of the skin, the dermis. After several hours the white frost gives way to a general pinkening, but it's the peeling off of the coagulated skin in the weeks afterward that gives the peel its name.

The best use of a deep phenol peel is to improve deep lines on the face, especially the deep lines around the mouth. For women with these particular type of wrinkles, lipstick is forever "bleeding" into these lip creases, making it impossible to have a clean lip line. Phenol is specifically toxic to the color-making cells of the skin (the melanocytes) and very often will permanently lighten the skin, sometimes making it look like a mottled marble cake. This lightening happens so often that patients need to be told up front—to improve their wrinkles, they must be ready to accept some color change in the skin.

Patient selection is everything with phenol. The ideal candidate is a very light-skinned, light-eyed person with deep wrinkles and facial liver spots who's willing to wear makeup at all times to cover up the possible change in skin color. After going through this selection process, there are not many left who should use phenol. Darker, olive-skinned patients are completely out of the question, since very often they heal with permanent lightening of the skin.

The skin is cleansed for all peels in the same way as for a dermabrasion. The use of an astringent such as rubbing alcohol or nail polish remover (acetone) to degrease the skin is even more important, as any remaining surface oil makes the penetration of any acid inconsistent. Phenol peels are quite painful and require IV sedation or even general anesthesia. There will also be pain following the peel.

Phenol is readily absorbed through the skin into your bloodstream and is toxic to the heart, so a constant heart monitor is very important during and after the surgery. People have actually died from phenol peels after the chemical buildup in the blood led to coma and death through this cardiac toxicity.

Once you have made it this far and the peel is done, you go into a recovery area for observation. Some doctors even apply tape over the skin that has been peeled so as to increase the penetration. After the tape is removed several days later, the skin will weep (water, or serum of the skin), and new skin will form to cover the wound in about seven days. Makeup may be applied in two to three weeks, and the redness and peeling of the skin subsides in the weeks afterward.

Why would anyone go through this? Prior to the introduction of the carbon dioxide laser, phenol was about the only way to really improve deep lip lines and deep crow's feet. Phenol gets the job done, but because of the need to select patients with light skin who are highly motivated to go through the pain and ordeal of the peel, the procedure is limited in its usefulness.

TCA (TRICHLOROACETIC ACID) PEELS

TCA is an acid that yields results that are in general not as dramatic as those produced by phenol, but the healing is quicker and less painful, there is no heart toxicity, and the mixture can be prepared in various levels of strength. For mild wrinkles, 20 to 30 percent strengths may be enough, while for deeper work,

35 to 50 percent may be needed. At this strength, most of the actual skin peeling occurs in the first four to seven days, and makeup may be worn at seven to fourteen days.

GLYCOLIC ACID PEELS

Derived from sugar cane, glycolic acid is part of a family of chemicals called alphahydroxy acids, and you may know it as the fruity acid peel. Glycolic has become enormously popular in the last few years, and it can even be bought without a prescription in a low concentration at any discount drugstore. It works in a small way; with long-term use, it will eventually improve the color irregularities of sun-damaged skin and even the earliest fine lines of younger people. After six months, the skin will usually have a healthy glow and generally look younger.

I think the best glycolic regimen is to start with a series of weekly peels done at a physician's office that progresses from 40 to 70 percent concentrations, as tolerated. These peels vary in cost around the country, but should be in the range of $50 to $70 each. At the same time you can start on a glycolic moisturizer and cleanser that can be continued at home for the long haul.

The procedure is done by applying the lotion on cleansed skin with a Q-tip or sponge. It is left on for anywhere between two and seven minutes, depending on your skin. The longer it is left on, the deeper the penetration ("deep" being a relative word since its penetration is shallow by definition). This reaction is stopped by rinsing the lotion off the skin with plain tap water; there is no frosting to be seen as with phenol or TCA. Glycolic acid cannot penetrate past the bottom of the epidermis. These peels are not painful and no anesthesia is needed—I have tried them and, at most, my skin tingled a bit. The next day the skin may be red and makeup can be worn, which is why glycolic acid is known as the "lunchtime face peel."

Complications of Dermabrasion and Phenol/TCA Peels

Both procedures present the distinct possibility of leaving the skin permanently lighter or darker, and the risk goes up significantly with olive- or darker-skinned patients. With phenol the lightening is so common that it shouldn't even be considered a complication as much as an unwanted byproduct. If the skin turns out darker, there are powerful bleach preparations containing the chemicals kojic acid or hydroquinone that can help lighten the tone. But if the skin turns out lighter, there's nothing to be done about it.

Other complications can include infection and, very rarely, the loss of the peeled skin. There is a wonderful medicine called Accutane, a pill to treat acne, which has the temporary side effect of making the skin dry. No resurfacing procedure should be done on anyone taking Accutane until its effects are long gone, usually at least a year.

A dreaded complication of any resurfacing procedure, including laser, is an outbreak of herpes simplex (cold sores) of the mouth or face. Normally a cold sore outbreak is confined to a small spot on the lip or skin. But when the skin is gone in the first week after any resurfacing procedure, the herpes virus is free to spread like wildfire to all the treated areas, and if this happens it would likely permanently scar the skin. To prevent this, I pretreat all resurfacing patients with a medicine called Zovirax.

About a year ago, I did a complete facial laser skin resurfacing on a beloved patient I had known for many years. In those days the standard was to give patients the Zovirax for several days before surgery and for one week after. This patient developed a herpes attack on the eighth postop day and it spread over her face rapidly and very painfully. I immediately restarted the Zovirax, which prevented any scarring. Cosmetic surgery is an unusually humbling business; every time you think you have seen it all, you see something you thought was impossible. I now routinely treat all postop resurfacing patients with Zovirax for two weeks.

In the first several months after any resurfacing surgery, it is possible that the new skin will form and heal too exuberantly, leading to a thickening and scarring that we call a keloid or a hypertrophic (thickened) scar. This can be treated belatedly by injecting dilute cortisone to erase the thickening, but better yet is for your doctor and staff to be alert for it and prevent it. In my postop followup appointments in the first two months after surgery, my staff or I will gently run our fingers over any persistently red areas and if the skin has the slightest firmness, I inject dilute cortisone to prevent this complication.

The Carbon Dioxide (CO_2) Laser

Lasers were first used in clinical medicine as early as 1962. These early machines put out a colored beam of light very much like those seen in *Star Wars* and were used to treat pigmented tumors of the skin and skin cancers. None were suited for cosmetic surgery because the laser light beam would, as a side effect, burn the skin and scar it. Though turning the skin into a charcoal briquette may be okay for treating a malignancy of the skin, I don't think it would be a popular or acceptable side effect for removing wrinkles or acne scars.

The first carbon dioxide lasers were invented in 1964 and first used clinically on people in 1967. These machines put out an invisible powerful beam of carbon dioxide but again were completely unsuitable for cosmetic surgery because of heat buildup and damage to the skin. The only solution would be to separate the light and heat, or at least minimize the heat buildup, so that no damage could be done.

The solution came decades later through two innovations: pulsing the light on and off and increasing its power greatly so that the energy needed for the laser to do its work could be delivered to the skin in a very short period. The most modern CO_2 lasers I use (the Coherent Corporation Ultrapulse) put out gigantic amounts of energy in a beam that pulses so rapidly that there is no heat buildup in your skin to harm it. In fact, the pulses of light are delivered so rapidly that any buildup of heat dissipates from the skin before the next pulse is delivered.

Modern CO_2 lasers are so remarkable that they've completely changed my notion of how to do cosmetic surgery. I simply no longer do any face peels or dermabrasions, and I no longer use a scalpel for eyelid lifts.

The powerful beam of carbon dioxide is absorbed by the water in the living cells of your skin. As the water absorbs the energy, the cell and skin are vaporized so rapidly that there is none of the heat buildup that could harm it. Because blood is really just a form of water, any bleeding at the skin's edge is also vaporized, so there is almost no bleeding. This makes laser safer for my patients than dermabrasion, phenol, or scalpel eyelid lifts. Because the CO_2 laser seals the nerve endings and lymphatics (which are responsible for swelling) as it works, it hurts less afterward and there is less swelling in recovery.

Remember earlier in the chapter when I complained that the frost seen in a peel and the blood flying in a dermabrasion make it hard for me to see exactly what I am doing? The laser has delightfully solved these problems. There is no frosting or bleeding at all, so the doctor can see exactly what he or she is doing and always knows the exact depth of the skin's layer as the procedure progresses.

In the sections on peel and dermabrasion I stress that these techniques are risky for olive- or darker-skinned people since the risk for permanent lightening or darkening is significant. I've treated people of every skin color with the CO_2 laser and have never seen a permanent color change in anyone; the machine is color blind. Sometimes people with very dark skin develop a temporary darkening about a month after a laser procedure, but in my experience this always resolves, and powerful bleaches can be used to make it resolve more quickly.

The machine has a keypad that can control every aspect of how the light is delivered: the power of the light beam (how hard it strikes the skin), the speed of the pulsing, the shape of the light, and even the overlap of the spots of light (density) are all infinitely controllable. That means that the thickness of skin vaporized in a single pass can be set so thin that the doctor at long last has an almost perfect control over the depth of the procedure. Whether I do the whole face or a single region, such as the mouth area, I do one pass at a time and evaluate my results and depth each time before I consider doing another pass. At the end of each finished pass, I wipe away the skin residue with a wet sponge to see exactly where I am and what I am doing. It is as if the skin were an onion with that typical wrinkled, thick oniony layer on the outside. With each pass of the laser I am removing about the thickness of a real single layer of onion skin until I reach that moist, soft, unwrinkled area below.

There are subtle color changes as, pass by pass, I go through the outer layer of the skin (the epidermis) and, layer by layer, enter the second layer of the skin (the dermis). After the first pass, when I have just gotten under the epidermis, the skin has a pink coloration to it. As I enter the dermis, the tissue has a light blue color. As I get deeper into the dermis the tissue turns yellow. When I have reached the part of the dermis where the tissue has a chamois yellow color, I stop whether the wrinkles are gone or not. This is because if I go deeper, the skin may have trouble healing properly and scar as a result. These color changes act as clear signposts to tell me exactly how deep I am, and this is where the experience and training of the doctor is everything. Sometimes I may need to do five or more passes to eliminate a deep lip wrinkle or improve a deep acne scar, but the beauty of using a laser is that each individual pass is so thin that there are many opportunities for evaluation and reflection before I find myself deeper than I would want to be.

The deeper you go, the greater the potential benefit, but also the more likely you are to have a poor healing, such as scar formation or permanent color change. With a perfect visual field and near perfect control of depth with the CO_2 laser, you can get the maximum benefit with the least risk of bad healing. It is a fantastic development in my field, and I'm thrilled to be able to use it on my patients.

The Procedure

After your skin is cleansed, anesthesia is achieved in several ways. If a single region is being resurfaced (such as the crow's feet around the eyes), an IV is used to give you a mild sedative and pain medication, while the skin is numbed with local anesthetic (Lidocaine). When the whole face is being treated, I sometimes block the large sensation nerves of the face and our anesthesiologist will give a deeper sedation through the IV. When a deep resurfacing is planned for severe wrinkles or acne scars, sometimes a modified general anesthesia is given, again by our resident anesthesiologist.

I first do one or two general passes over the areas to be treated so as to remove all the old skin. Magically a lifetime of sun damage, liver spots, and pigment irregularity are wiped away. But, at this stage, I have not yet gone deep enough to improve the wrinkles or scars that extend much deeper into the dermis, so I then change the tip on the laser that focuses and directs the light beam and methodically work out the wrinkles or scars. The light can be shaped like a circle, a triangle, square, or even a rectangle. This is very useful because all scars and wrinkles have different contours, and I can shape the light to best improve the problem.

At the end of the procedure there is no bleeding, but the skin is pretty raw, and I protect it with either a dressing, a clean bandage, or a layer of antibiotic ointment heavily applied to the skin. After the surgery is over the patient goes to a specially equipped recovery area under the direction of experienced, specialized recovery nurses. After several hours of monitoring, all of my patients go home to sleep in their own beds.

Afterward

I have people return the very next day (even on Saturday) for a checkup. No matter how much I prepare people at the consultation or how many times I tell them on the morning of surgery about how bad it will look the next day, people are still worried and always have an extreme case of buyer's remorse. The skin is red, weepy, and looks just like you stepped out of central casting for a *Nightmare on Elm Street* movie, but over the following two weeks the skin steadily improves, the weeping stops after five or six days, and the support and assurance given by myself and my fabulous nurses gets you through this. Strangely enough, laser resurfacing usually hurts very little afterward. Most people say it feels like a mild, stinging sunburn. One of my patients, Shirley, described it this way:

> Believe it or not, the first cosmetic surgery I ever had was when Dr. Gaynor did my eyes with his laser on national television. It was just amazing, because I felt nothing at all during the operation and only the slightest tickle, like a very mild sunburn, afterward, and the results were terrific. I had gone to him because of the great work he'd done for my daughter, Jayne, and I was so happy with what he did for me that I went back and had a complete and serious facial resurfacing, during which there was also no sensation. Afterward, though, my face swelled up and I looked like the moon, there was a discomfort like a serious sunburn for about a week, and I kept thinking "What have I done?" But after about five days or so, I was back to normal—except I looked at least ten years younger. Everyone talks about how

rested I look and what a glow I have—but they have no idea I had work done. It's that subtle.

The Results

When people first see that every wrinkle and scar is gone, they get very excited. Unfortunately, this is an illusion caused by the postop swelling stretching the skin. After the swelling starts to go down, some of the wrinkles and scars return partly, but they are still better than before surgery, and this benefit is the real McCoy. Yet it isn't as good as you expected, and practically everyone falls into an emotional trough during this phase, since the skin is still fire engine red from healing.

The very vivid redness of the healing phase slowly tones down, although some redness may stay for three or four months. A key element in the recovery of patients from any resurfacing technique is to use camouflage makeup after two weeks to hide the redness. Our staff includes a makeup artist who's responsible for getting the postlaser patient back to work and out on the town. The artist will look at your original skin tone and the amount of laser work that's been done to pick your skin's opposite color on the color wheel. If you're a blond, for example, and your face postlaser is the typical beet red, you'll actually be daubed with green makeup! The combination of your red skin with just the right hint of green is, believe it or not, a natural-looking skin color, which can then be touched over with foundation so as to make a normal appearance; it works well even for men who have to go back to work.

The great magic of the carbon dioxide laser occurs from the second to the fourth month after the surgery. Scars and wrinkles get better and better until there is usually a tremendous improvement over the original. What is happening is that the skin is actually tightening from the harmless heat that was emitted by the laser. The underlying connective tissue of the skin is shrinking and tightening the skin itself. Another fabulous change occurs to the feel of the skin, which slowly softens in the months after laser surgery until it feels like the legendary baby's bottom. This softness will stay for many years, especially if you've stopped trying to tan.

The Erbium Laser

The new erbium lasers put out a beam of light that is also absorbed by the water in living skin, but the depth of penetration is less than that of the CO_2. A good rule of thumb is that it takes two or three passes with the erbium to equal the depth of a single pass with the CO_2. Though this technology is just beginning to be understood, I feel this machine benefits completely different people than the CO_2 laser.

Especially in fair-skinned people, there can be a great deal of sun damage and pigment change in the outer layer of the skin, accompanied by the first signs of crow's feet and lip wrinkles. Though you can use the CO_2 laser at very low levels to laser away this problem, it's a little like driving a Porsche cross-country in first gear. The erbium laser is only meant to be absorbed by the superficial skin and will likely turn out to be the better machine to treat all people when the goal is to polish the outer layer only. Recovery is just a few days, and the price will likely be a fraction of that charged for a full-face deep CO_2 resurfacing. What's really exciting is that the erbium laser shows great potential for reducing wrinkles in the lower neck and on the backs of the hands, two areas that have not benefited from the magic of cosmetic surgery before now.

The Cost

The cost of all resurfacing techniques ranges widely depending on whether you do a small or large single area, several areas, or the whole face. Most doctors charge less to do shallow wrinkles and scars than deep ones. A single area, such as crow's feet, may cost somewhere between $1,000 and $2,500, while the whole face can cost more than $7,000.

FREQUENTLY ASKED QUESTIONS

When can I go out in the sun after laser skin resurfacing?

Parents know to put sun hats on brand new babies, and the same attitude applies to your new skin, which can be very easily damaged by direct exposure to the sun. This especially applies to darker skinned people where direct sun damage in the first few months may lead to a very stubborn darkening that is very difficult to bleach.

I usually tell patients to avoid all direct sun exposure for at least three months. This doesn't mean that our patients can only go out after sundown or are forced to walk next to tall buildings on the shady side of the street. There are wonderful, powerful sunscreens that offer great protection, as well as a wonderful range of styles in wide-brimmed hats.

When can I go back to work?

Because the laser is infinitely programmable, each person has a unique recovery. For people who have resurfacing for early signs of skin aging such as light liver spots and fine wrinkles, camouflage makeup can often be applied after about a week, and they can return to work then. When people have deep wrinkles or scars, the skin will take two weeks or longer to heal well enough to apply camouflage and go back to work.

In my practice men and women have laser resurfacing in equal numbers, and my cosmetologist teaches the men to apply the camouflage just like the women. When applied well, it is almost impossible to detect. After three weeks you will still look very red, but you can get away with saying it's a sunburn or that you fell asleep in your favorite tanning parlor.

When will my skin look good without makeup?

By the third or fourth week the skin looks like a moderate pink sunburn, which will remain for about three to four months.

How much improvement can I expect with laser skin resurfacing?

The laser produces a greater degree of correction of wrinkles and scars than does dermabrasion and peel. For acne scars, the dermabrasion will produce roughly a 30 to 40 percent improvement, while with laser, 60 to 80 percent is not unusual. For wrinkles, phenol peels can be as effective as the laser, but afterward the skin is often permanently lighter, and the surface loses its normal markings and can take on an alabaster look. When the laser improves wrinkles, it puts life and softness back into the skin, a great advantage.

Chapter 8

✳

CAN YOU SAY *BLEPHAROPLASTY*?

THE EYELID LIFT

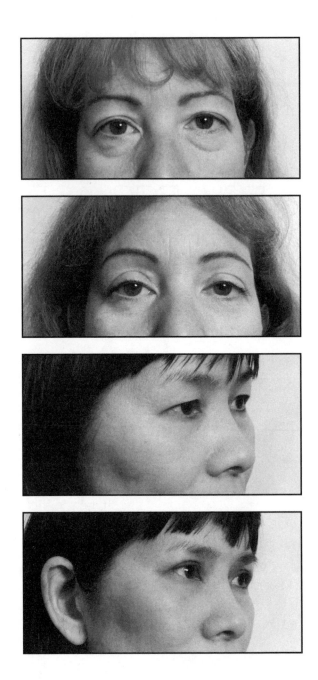

(above) CO₂ Laser Upper and Lower Eyelid Lift—before and after
(below) CO₂ Laser Upper Eyelid Lift—before and after

140

In almost all human encounters we look into each other's eyes and that moment is our first (and frequently longest-lasting) impression. Nothing makes human beings look older than sagging, loose, and wrinkly skin around the eyes accompanied by bulges of fat—the hallmarks that a lid lift should be seriously considered. Women always know when it's time, since the aged upper eyelid skin becomes so loose it gets difficult to wear makeup. I've even seen men and women come into my office where the upper eyelid skin is actually resting on the eyelashes and can interfere with peripheral vision.

Heavy lower eyelids tend to run in my family. By the time we reach our twenties and thirties we always look tired, no matter how much sleep we've gotten. I remember that my father always looked tired to me even when I was very young, because of his huge lower lid fat bags. I had my own lower lids done in 1985, and in 1997, my twenty-one-year-old daughter, Beth, asked me to do her lids as well, since all her friends at college were telling her *she* always looked tired. I did it even though, as an adoring father, she looked perfect to me.

One of my patients, Marie De Martini, also had the family curse of baggy lower lids, and before she came to see me, she remembered trying to fix it with

> cucumbers and ice cubes, but nothing would reduce the puffiness and everyone always telling me how tired I looked. Finally I turned sixty-five and thought, enough is enough, and had the work done, and couldn't believe I'd waited so long. Everyone was suddenly saying "You look great!" and "What have you been doing to yourself?" The whole thing was so great that now I'm saving up for a minilift, and I tell all my friends, you owe it to yourself to look good if you can.

After a certain age, though, it isn't just genetics; all of us can benefit from eyelid work. Because of some innovative new techniques, right now is a very exciting time for someone like me to do eyelid surgery. Upper and lower lifts can be done together or separately, depending on your preference, need, and budget. A successful, totally customized lid lift produces a change that is one of the most satisfying in all of cosmetic surgery.

Upper Eyelid Lift

The purpose here is to remove loose, wrinkly skin and the bulges of extra fat. The first step is to make a blueprint with ink of the skin to be removed so as to guide the surgeon's work. It's key to do this when someone is sitting upright so as to note the effect of gravity pulling on the skin. It is everything in upper eyelid surgery to mark exactly the right amount of skin to be removed, since if too little is taken out the change is not as dramatic as it should be and if too much is removed you get the dreadful complication of not being able to close the eye.

The next step is to apply antiseptic and numb the skin with local anesthetic (Lidocaine). Frequently, patients also want IV sedation to relax and make the time go quickly. The extra skin and fat responsible for the old look are then removed, either with a scalpel or laser, and the gap in the skin is sewn with very thin suture. Believe it or not, the upper eyelids have two bags of fat that must be removed, and each is as large as a piece of popped popcorn (or pickled pepper). I always try to take a Polaroid of these bags to show patients the next day at their checkup since they always say exactly the same thing: "That couldn't have been in my eyes!" The patient rests for several hours in the recovery area and can then go home with some help from a friend or loved one.

In my own practice I use the laser to do eyelid lifts, and here's why: When surgeons use a scalpel, they rely on the sensation of touch transmitted from the blade touching the patient's skin through the scalpel handle to their hand to know if they are applying the correct amount of pressure. Factors such as the time of the day, the sharpness of the blade (not all scalpel blades are created equally at the factory), the amount of caffeine in the espresso or cola your doctor had prior to surgery . . . all can make a difference.

With a CO_2 laser, however, there is no possibility of variability of pressure, and the laser never even touches the skin; it's held several inches away. Because the actual energy of the laser is programmed in by the doctor through a keypad, when the pulse of light is delivered it will always have the exact force programmed in beforehand, the setting of which is determined by the experience of the surgeon, with a scientific control that is wonderful and reliable. Additionally, there is much less bleeding with a laser, and I think that the bruising is less, and the postop healing faster. I loved doing scalpel surgery in the past, but I'll never go back and do it that way again.

Lower Eyelid Lift

If friends are constantly telling you how tired you look all the time, it's because of fat bags in the lower eyelids, and you'll greatly benefit from a lower eyelid lift. The prepping of the skin and antiseptic scrub are the same as are used for upper lids. For lower eyelids the marking is not nearly as important because, depending on the method, little if any skin is removed.

There are two ways to get at the fat. In one method the skin is opened just below the eyelash line with a scalpel, the bags of fat are teased out through the incision, and depending on your original problem, little or no actual skin is removed; then the gap is sewn with fine suture. In the other method, the fat is teased out through the inside wet skin (conjunctiva) of the eyelid, and no sewing is needed because that skin heals wonderfully all by itself. When the surgery is done, you go to the recovery area for rest and monitoring, and then go home.

When I had the fat removed from my lower eyelids about fifteen years ago, there were no lasers available for cosmetic surgery and the method of removing the fat bags through the inside of the skin hadn't been developed yet, so the fat was taken through a tiny scalpel incision just below the lower eyelashes. The scar healed beautifully and imperceptibly, and in general the work was superbly done. Yet there was a very subtle change afterward in the shape of my eyes—they were a bit rounder than before. Most of us naturally have an almond shape to our eyes, something we may not value until it's gone. For me, the slight rounding created a more open-eyed, sadder look.

Because injured skin tends to shrink as it heals, the scar line of your eyelid lift will slightly shrink in the six months after surgery. This shrinkage of the scar is what causes the lower eyelid to slightly drop, resulting in the rounder, sadder look. It has nothing to do with the skill of your surgeon; it can happen to anyone. I used to tell people at consultations of this likely shape change in the eyes, and almost without exception it made no difference to them. But, after I switched to removing the fat from lower eyelids through the inside, eye rounding became a thing of the past.

This is why almost without exception I use my CO_2 laser to make a small opening in the lower eyelid skin from the inside (the conjunctiva side). Through that incision I tease out the three bags of fat. Because the outside skin is never touched, it has little if any reason to shrink.

The Preparation

At the consultation I take a thorough history, screening for any preexisting illnesses (such as heart disease, diabetes, or high blood pressure) that could effect the surgery's outcome. It's not that people with these problems can't have an eyelid lift, it's just that they need to have these problems under good control and managed by their family doctor before the surgery. Routine blood tests will check for hidden anemia and the rate of clotting.

It is very important before an eyelid lift to have an eye exam to check your vision, ability to make tears, and other ocular functions. (Some doctors charge so much for eye surgery that quoting their fee is in itself a test of their patient's ability to make tears.) It's critical that all patients be off aspirin, or aspirin-containing products, and alcohol for two weeks prior to surgery. These products greatly increase bleeding in surgery and can make the surgery so much more dangerous that people have actually gone blind from an eyelid lift.

The Procedure

Eyelid lifts are an outpatient procedure that can be done in a well-equipped operating room in your doctor's office or even in the new outpatient surgicenters of your local hospital. The lift takes little more than an hour, and with the combination of local anesthesia (Lidocaine) and IV sedation, it should be an easy and pain-free experience for the patient. After the surgery the patient is observed in a recovery area by a nurse and is then sent home. The whole time spent in the clinic is four to six hours, though this can vary.

Afterward

For the first few nights after surgery, I have people sleep as upright as possible to minimize postop bleeding. It's crucial to apply ice packs or bags of frozen peas to the eyes on and off for the first two or three days to minimize swelling and bruising. Patients are sent home with pain medication and antibiotics, as well as a few sleeping pills like Valium. There is seldom much pain afterward, but trying to sleep upright is almost impossible without the sleeping pills. In fact, if you have severe pain afterward in the eye itself, you should call your doctor immediately, as this can be a sign of a severe complication.

For two weeks, no heavy exertion is allowed—no lifting, no working out, and no squabbling. Anything that increases blood pressure will increase swelling and bruising and might even lead to the type of bleeding that can cause blindness.

In my experience, men are apt to break this rule much more than women. Recently I was called out of surgery to see a man who'd had an eyelid lift two days before, and he now had the most bruised and swollen eyelids I'd ever seen. After checking carefully I was relieved to see that his vision was normal and that there was no unusual bleeding, but I'd never had any lid patient before with such an appearance. Finally he admitted that he'd done a full stationary bike aerobic workout the morning after surgery. It was his routine, and he wasn't going to be a "sissy" and skip it, just because he'd had surgery.

The Results

Stitches come out in a week or less. By the end of the first week the obvious swelling and bruising is usually gone and you can be seen without sunglasses. After the stitches are removed, women can wear makeup and most can go back to work without anyone noticing. You'll begin to see the benefit within two to three weeks, and the improvement will get better and better for up to six months as the healing progresses.

Complications

Infections can occur after any surgery, but they are not common after blepharoplasty; other complications can occur when too much skin is removed, making it difficult or impossible to close the eyelids fully. Too much fat removal can give you a hollow, gaunt look and is unfortunately not rare. In traditional lower lifts with a skin incision, the skin may shrink enough so that you see the white part of the eye under the iris—not a good look. There's also the possibility of an ectropion, which is a pulling down of the lower eyelid that is so severe that the skin is no longer in contact with the eyeball. This requires a complex repair or even several procedures to correct.

The most dreaded complication of an eyelid lift is a decrease in vision or even blindness, but thank goodness, this is extremely rare. If, in the first few days after the procedure, you suddenly develop severe pain around or behind the eye, call your doctor immediately. This pain may be from a small amount of blood accumulating behind the eye that applies pressure to the eyeball and could damage your vision.

The Costs

Fees for eyelid lifts can be quoted "by the lid" (uppers or lowers) or for all four lids. Fees vary enormously, and the best way for you to determine the customary range of fees where you live is to call a few highly recommended doctors specializing in eyelid surgery; a reference from a friend who had a good result is hard to beat. All-fours can range in price from $3,000 to $8,000, and more often than not, the fee for all four is usually less than doing the lids on separate days. For example, a surgeon may charge $2,000 to do uppers or lowers, but charge $3,500 if all four are done at once.

FREQUENTLY ASKED QUESTIONS

How long does an eyelid lift last?

This varies enormously, but benefits of ten years or longer are common. If you look in a mirror and blink, you'll see that the upper eyelids do most of the work, so this skin will loosen eventually. In the past, when the skin loosened, the way to fix it was to do another lift, but now I can simply numb the upper eyelid and resurface the skin using my laser; this usually shrinks the skin enough to work.

Will the fat bags come back?

I've never seen the fat bags come back, but I have seen the lower lids bulge again years later, making people look tired. How is this possible?

When I remove fat from the lower lids, I'm walking a fine line—too much, and you'll have that gaunt, hollow look of a cadaver. But if I remove too little, the benefit is inadequate, and I will have to go back and take more. I've seen so many patients in consultation who have the hollow look of an overzealous lid job that I try to avoid it at all costs (fortunately, it's never happened to one of my patients). Sometimes, especially in younger patients, I intentionally leave a little lower eyelid fat behind to avoid any possibility of overdoing it. Now, of course, we can use the fat transfer method to fix other doctors' miscalculations.

So the answer to the question is that, if I or any surgeon errs too far on the side of safety, later on in life you may again have tired-looking lids.

Will my eyelid wrinkles and crow's feet improve with an eyelid lift?

No. Almost every patient in consultation thinks the lift will automatically take care of wrinkles and crow's feet, but these are textural problems that can only be improved by resurfacing with a peel or laser.

Chapter 9

YOUR FACE

FACELIFTS, BROWLIFTS, AND ALTERNATIVE FACIAL SURGERY

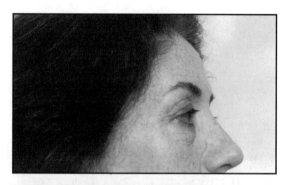

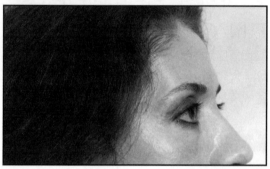

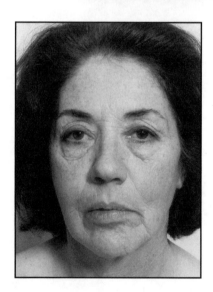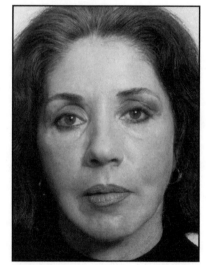

Mini Brow Lift, CO_2 Laser Upper and Lower Eyelid Lift,
CO_2 Laser Skin Resurfacing—before and after

For many cosmetic surgeons, fixing an aging face represents the heart and soul of why they chose their careers. If the goal of all cosmetic surgery is to improve the appearance, reverse the signs of aging, and give the patient a better outlook, nothing can beat the superbly done facelift. So many of my patients come in for consultations with such tired and droopy looks that it's only after they've had their facelifts that I realize how attractive they were in the first place.

I had my own mini-facelift three years ago, and every time someone I haven't seen in a while tells me how rested I look or that I've never looked better, I get the same emotional lift that patients tell me makes their experience so worthwhile.

How do you know if you'd benefit from a lift? Look at your face in a mirror, starting with the forehead. Do you have horizontal wrinkles that are just beginning to show, or are they so deeply grooved into the skin you look like a woodworking experiment? Do you have vertical lines between the eyebrows that make you look angry all the time, or horizontal lines on the top of the nose where it meets the forehead?

For the women reading this book, if you have been tweezing your eyebrows ever more vigorously over the years, or using a pencil to create a high, arched look to compensate for the effects of gravity, you know you could benefit from a browlift. The change in the shape of the eyebrow from aging and gravity, causing it to flatten and fall, can alter the whole expression of your face from a happy one to a sad, angry, or tired look.

Now look at the furrows that go from the nostril of the nose to the corners of the mouth, the laugh lines. Are they heavier and deeper than they used to be? If there's a fullness and heaviness to the face just outside these lines, chances are that the cheek fat pouch (that made you look fine when it was where it belonged, higher up on the face) has migrated downward, making you look heavy and hangdog.

My patients tell me that the marionette, or puppet, lines that go from the corner of the mouth to the chin on both sides are the wrinkles that bother them the most. Drooping puppet lines and deep laugh lines give the whole mouth and lower face a turned-down, unhappy look.

Next, consider the jawline as it extends from the chin to the ears. Do you have a squirrel pouch there that marks the onset of jowls? And, below the jaw, do you have the cords and hanging skin that typify the turkey neck?

If any or all of these signs of aging are present, don't get mad or upset. All of them can now be fixed with new methods of cosmetic surgery that make it more practical, safe, and appealing than ever before. The facelift, the browlift, and the alternative facelift can all reverse the effects of gravity. If you have crow's feet around the eyes, deep lines around the lips, scars from acne and chicken pox, or liver and sunspots on your face, no lift will improve them; you'll need a resurfacing. But if your looks have declined because of the aging effects of gravity, this is the chapter for you.

The Aesthetics of the Face

Every artist who learns to draw the human face learns that the most beautiful and harmonious heads are roughly divided into thirds, with the spaces from the hairline to the top of the nose, from the top of the nose to tip of the nose, and from the tip of the nose to the tip of the chin being about equal. Many of the changes seen in aging distort these fine proportions. For example, when a man is balding with a receding hairline, the forehead becomes far more than one-third the length of the face. When the turkey gobbler neck starts to hang down, it makes the lower part of the face seem too long. The artful cosmetic surgeon restores these harmonious proportions and helps patients once again achieve the classic symmetry of youth.

The Classic Facelift

Many doctors have taught me their facelift techniques and philosophies, but the teacher from whom I've learned the most is Dr. Alberto Hodara, an extraordinary plastic surgeon working in Porto Alegre, Brazil. I think many of you are wondering: Why Brazil? With so many extraordinary surgeons in America, why go there?

In fact, the roots of the facelift come directly from Brazil. Dr. Ivo Pitungay of Rio de Janeiro is the father of the original, modern facelift, and he began a Brazilian aesthetic for cosmetic surgery that achieves completely natural results. The finest American surgeons now, of course, all feel the same way, but watching the Academy Awards with all those famous folk (whose faces look like they've been left in a wind tunnel for forty-eight hours) tells me that some surgeons still just don't know when to stop.

The Procedure

The facelift may be done under local anesthetic with Lidocaine and IV sedation to relax the patient, or under general anesthesia. My mini-facelift was done under local anesthesia, and that's what I prefer for my patients.

The marking of the facial areas is very important, very much as a carefully drawn blueprint would be to an architect, but no two doctors do these exactly alike and no one method is more valid than any other method, as long as it safely and reliably produces the results you want.

The face and whole top of the head are washed with an antiseptic liquid. The hair is pinned up with sterile tin foil to keep it from getting in the way; I never cut the hair when doing a facelift. The incision lines and the whole pocket area where the skin is to be undermined are numbed with a dilute solution of local anesthetic. The IV sedation makes this a very happy twilight kind of experience.

I have been blessed by the great surgeons who have taken me under their wings. When I was first learning to do facelifts, Dr. Hodara would stand directly across the table to observe and supervise my work while Dr. Remo Farina, also a plastic surgeon, would stand just to my right to look under the skin as I worked to make sure I was just where I should be. The intense and personal training they gave me over an extended period of time is always with me when I operate.

After the outlines are cut and the tissue loosened, the skin can slide over the underlying deeper tissue and be pulled in an upward direction—the lift—to reverse the droopy look of gravity that made a facelift desirable in the first place. It's exactly like making a bed and pulling up the rumpled blanket to make everything look neat and tidy. This is where technique and science end, and art and judgment are everything. How much pull is enough? How much is too much?

I know that for a patient to consider a facelift successful, a key issue is to get as much improvement in the laugh and puppet lines as possible; everyone says that. The actual pull in a facelift goes in the general direction of a straight line that would go from the tip of the nose to the top of the ear. If you look in the mirror and grasp the skin just in front of the top of your ear and pull backward and upward along this line, you will see at first a lovely improvement in the droop in the center of the face, but if you keep pulling, something very different happens. Watch the mouth and lips; they'll start to move as well. If you now pull from both sides, you will see that awful windswept look that characterizes an overdone lift. You might now be ready to announce Oscar nominations, but you won't get this look from me.

When I actually get to the lifting part of the facelift, I pull until I see the slightest movement of the mouth, and then I back off about 10 percent. I do this several times to be sure and then mark the skin to be removed. Sometimes potential patients who consult with me want so much pull that even a permanent grimace to the mouth would not deter them. They are not wrong. People should get what they want if they understand all the facts. But they will never convince me to be their doctor, because to perform the surgery the way they want it would violate the most sacred rule of surgery for me and the teachers whose thoughts and values go through my head whenever I do surgery: All surgery must produce a completely natural result and never call attention to itself. My patients and I can never hear too many compliments about how rested, youthful, and wonderful we look. But I would be embarrassed beyond belief if any patient I operated on was told by a friend, "Well, you finally did your face!" This is no compliment.

Once I have marked the skin, all the extra skin is then trimmed off, and the incision sites are closed with stitches. For most of my mini-procedures, I use no formal bandage but many doctors wrap the head in a babushka-type bandage for several days.

SMAS, Extended SMAS, and Composite Facelifts

The classic facelift I have just described is really a skin/fat lift, because there is no attempt to manipulate deeper tissues such as the facial muscles. There are distinct limitations to the classic skin/fat lift. For one thing, the benefit obtained in improving the aging in the central part of the face, particularly the laugh lines, the puppet lines, and the descending cheek fat pads, is almost always less than the improvement seen in the jowls and the turkey neck. Even worse is that, for most of us, the earliest changes we notice, even in our thirties and forties, as our faces age are not caused by the stretching of the skin and so can't be fully fixed by lifting the skin. This is particularly true of horizontal forehead wrinkles, early flattening and drooping of the eyebrow, and the deepening of the vertical lines between the eyebrows, the laugh lines, and the puppet lines. These changes are more often than not caused by the relaxation of deeper muscles and other tissues, and so can only be partly corrected by the traditional facelift I described above. It was logical for doctors to develop new kinds of facelifts to address these deeper causes of aging.

You should know that the value (and even the validity) of these deeper facelifts is being fought over right now at medical meetings and in medical journals. I'll explain my own opinion, but remember that very committed and smart doctors are passionately arguing about such issues and the future direction of facelifts.

The SMAS (superficial musculoaponeurotic system) facelift was first reported in the medical literature in 1976. The name SMAS is more daunting than the lift itself. The idea is that, instead of lifting the skin and fat only, a two-level facelift is performed that lifts the superficial muscles under the skin as well as the skin itself. In 1977, a study was done in which more than twenty patients agreed to have half of their face lifted with the traditional facelift and the other side done with the SMAS lift, all on the same day (talk about patient trust—I would not want to ask my patients to have two different lifts done at the same time). Happily for these patients, it made no difference at all. This study definitively showed that the SMAS side was not more dramatically helped than the other and that the benefit lasted no longer. Several other studies carried out over the ensuing years also concluded that SMAS was neither more beneficial nor longer lasting, but the risk was definitely not the same: the deeper the facelift, the more exposed the crucial nerves of the face, and the greater the risk of nerve injury.

In the last ten years, several even deeper and more aggressive facelifts have been invented, including the extended SMAS and, the deepest yet, the composite facelift. In the composite, the surgeon is so deeply into the substance of the face that the most important nerve, the facial nerve itself, which is very easily injured, is often exposed, as it is right in the field where the surgeon is working. In 1996, another study was reported that looked at the results of more than twenty people who, like the volunteers in 1977, had had different types of lifts done on the halves of their face on the same day. Some had regular SMAS on one side, extended SMAS on the other, while others had extended SMAS on one side and composite facelifts on the other. I bet you can guess the outcome of this study. No difference in benefit was seen, no matter which method was used.

The deeper lifts, however, do have a price. As many as 0.8 percent of people getting the deepest lifts have some form of temporary facial paralysis, and for 0.1 percent (one in one thousand), the paralysis is permanent. This is an astonishingly high rate of injury for a procedure that has yet to be shown to be of any real or lasting benefit. These deeper lifts also require much longer recovery times and patients experience extended swelling and numbness.

Now I know that some doctors disagree with these findings, and in fact there was a very strong rebuttal to this report in the same journal. But I feel so strongly about these studies that I have noted the article describing them in the bibliography for your reference. Don't let your doctor do any more than a skin-lift on you unless he or she is familiar with this study and can explain to you, in terms you understand, why you should have a multilevel lift. Most medical libraries have open stacks with periodicals where anyone can browse without charge. The introduction and conclusion to this important paper are written in a clear English that you can understand.

The Browlift

If you have a drooping in the shape of the eyebrows that makes you look sad, angry, or tired, or a hooding of loose skin just above the outer part of the eye itself, or deep horizontal forehead wrinkles, or vertical furrows between the eyebrows, the browlift may be for you. The browlift can be done partially (a mini-browlift corrects the hooding only) or the whole brow can be lifted (the coronal browlift).

CORONAL BROWLIFT

The coronal browlift can be done under local anesthesia with IV sedation or general anesthesia. The incision goes from ear to ear on top of the head behind the hairline, so it's unfortunately not suitable for men who are balding and have unstable hairlines or for women with thin hair.

After the anesthesia has taken effect, the skin is incised and then loosened. The loose skin is pulled back, the extra skin is trimmed, and the suture line is either sewn or stapled. This whole procedure usually takes less than an hour, and when it is done well, the eyebrow shape improves, the horizontal lines improve, and even the vertical lines that make people look angry are frequently eliminated.

So, what's wrong with this picture? Unfortunately, the coronal lift has many limitations. For one, it stretches and widens the width of the forehead relative to the hairline. If your forehead is relatively wide naturally, this increase in width will distort the harmonious rule of thirds and throw the face out of balance. The nerves for sensation to the top of the head run through the scalp and are cut with the incision, and for many people, there is temporary or permanent numbness on the top of the head. Such numbness won't shorten anyone's life, but it is irritating, especially when it lasts forever. Finally, some people have permanent hair loss along the scar line that shows as a white, bald, thin line that can be seen, especially when the wind is blowing. I am not saying the procedure is bad in general, but there are so many problems that I seldom offer it to anyone.

ENDOSCOPIC BROWLIFT

For younger people, who are just beginning to see the signs of brow problems, the coronal browlift would be like using a sledgehammer to kill a fly. Instead, an endoscope, a narrow tube with a bright light on the end that is placed under the skin, is used to see inside. The endoscopic technique can improve drooping brow and forehead wrinkles (caused by the relaxation of deeper tissues) by directly working under the skin where the benefit is needed, sidestepping the worst side effects of coronal browlift. It can be done under local anesthetic (Lidocaine) with IV sedation or under general anesthesia.

Usually there are five small (less than one inch each) incisions made just behind the hairline in a front to back orientation. The forehead skin is then pulled up and tacked down to the deeper tissue, and as unbelievable as it sounds, the forehead skin will adhere in this higher position as part of the natural healing process. There may be a small hump of skin for a short time, but the skin will naturally redistribute itself, eliminating the hump. The small incisions are sewn and usually heal with no visible scarring.

Alternative Facial Surgery

The facelifts and browlifts described above are large surgeries that can correct several problems at once, but they can also leave highly visible scars and often require lengthy recoveries. I've found that many people are afraid of such large-scale procedures or can't afford them or don't want to live with the hairstyle sometimes needed to hide the scars. In fact, for men with short or thin hair, it's impossible to have a full-blown facelift or browlift.

In alternative facial surgery, the goal is to listen to the patient's concerns and find a small-scale procedure that solves the problem without getting carried away. If someone comes in and is worried about a turkey neck, why lift the face or the brow? If another person is only worried about the brow, why lift the neck? Now, of course, I haven't thrown out all traditional surgery, and in fact some procedures like partial browlift (I call this a minibrow) are still very useful. But by replacing older, bulky techniques with smaller, simpler, less expensive ones, alternative facial surgery can offer you a variety of choices never before possible.

At the start of this chapter are a few before-and-after sets of one alternative surgery patient, Lucretia. To accomplish this in the past, she would've needed:

- a full lower facelift and complete coronal browlift;
- a scalpel upper and lower eyelid lift;

- a deep chemical peel; and
- collagen injections.

Instead, we began by using what I call a mini-browlift to improve the droopy hooding in the outside of her eyebrow. In the minibrow, a small incision is made above the top of the ear, well behind the hairline, and is extended in a semicircular arc several inches upward. After undermining the skin and pulling it backward, the extra skin can be trimmed off and sewn in a one-hour surgery that requires no formal bandage. But wait—the minibrow only fixes the brow, not the horizontal or vertical wrinkles. Yet, look closely and you'll see that the wrinkles and brow position on her forehead are much improved as well. I used the CO_2 laser to resurface the worn-out skin on her entire face. The laser retextures old skin and moderately tightens it as well. This combination of mini-browlift and forehead laser resurfacing can replace the big browlift for almost everyone. To finish off the upper third of her face, I took a little fat from her lower body to fill in the vertical forehead lines and to plump up the laugh and puppet lines.

Lucretia's upper and lower eyelid lifts were done with the laser, while a minituck dramatically improved her laugh lines, puppet lines, and jowls. The minituck is done with an incision line that only extends from the top to the bottom of the ear in its natural crease.

Finally, I did some liposculpture on the fat pads just outside her laugh lines to reduce the heavy, droopy look of the central part of the face, a procedure that can be used instead of the composite facelift.

How long did it take for Lucretia to have all this surgery? One day. And the change in everything about her was remarkable. She went for a whole new wardrobe, a whole new hair and makeup look, and a whole new attitude. Seeing her after the surgery was like seeing a woman who'd been made young all over again, and every day was her birthday.

Another of my patients, Jayne, was so happy with the results of her liposuction that she learned all about the latest advances in cosmetic surgery, and said, "I love that now you can do mini-procedures and just keep looking great your whole life. That's the philosophy I'm going to live by—to keep everything maintained and never let anything go. I'll nip and tuck all the way to the grave!"

The Preparation

All patients are required to have blood tests prior to surgery to make sure blood counts are normal and that there is no underlying bleeding tendency. If the patient is older, sometimes an EKG, a chest X-ray, and perhaps a note from a family doctor will be needed before I will go ahead. If patients have diabetes, high blood pressure, or other illnesses, most of them can still go ahead with surgery if these conditions are under good control. All aspirin and aspirin-containing products (cold remedies, for example) need to have been stopped at least two weeks prior to surgery because they can interfere with clotting and healing.

More so than with any other kind of cosmetic surgery, it is most critical that you stop smoking at least two weeks before any facelift and not start again for at least several weeks afterward. Smoking so hampers blood supply to the healing skin that you can actually lose massive patches of skin, which will lead to catastrophic scarring.

The Procedure

After signing the consent forms, getting preop pictures taken, and completing payment for the surgery (if you haven't paid in advance), the patient will change into a paper gown and any makeup will be removed. I then carefully mark the surgical areas so as to create a perfect blueprint to follow as I operate. These surgeries can take anywhere from one to six hours, depending on how much work is being done, but the patient feels no pain or anxiety.

Afterward

A trained recovery room nurse will monitor the patient in a specially equipped recovery area. Our nurses will not let patients leave until they are stable and the time is right. How long are you likely to be at the office? Most of the day. My patients are usually ready to leave about three to five hours after the surgery, even when they've had multiple procedures. Someone must be available to take them home.

In large lifts there are usually bandages placed around the face and head for one or two days. People are really glad when these are removed. In all my minilifts, I use no formal bandages at all, and I even let people shower within one or two days.

In facial surgery it is very important to really take it easy for the first two weeks following surgery. I try to get the patients to sleep either in recliner chairs that are almost upright or on several pillows in bed, so there's no increased blood pressure from having the head lower than the heart. The increased blood pressure of just lying down flat can lead to accumulation of blood under the skin, forming a hematoma that could disastrously effect the outcome. The hematoma can stretch and put pressure on the loosened skin in a way that cuts off its blood supply, leading to a total loss of a large area of the skin. Hematoma problems are far less likely to happen after a minilift because there is much less undermined tissue.

In large facelifts, bruising and swelling last about two weeks or less. In deep SMAS and composite lifts, swelling can go on for months. In my minilifts, bruising and swelling are less common and resolve usually in three or four days. Many out-of-town patients who have these procedures actually go sightseeing in San Francisco within one or two days after a minilift.

I ask most of my patients to take one or two weeks off work to relax and set this time aside in their lives to devote to healing and recovery. Since almost all patients with minilifts are out and about within a day or two, this can be a very enjoyable time. I give all patients a week of antibiotics, let them shampoo and shower within several days, and remove all stitches between the seventh and fourteenth day.

The Results

People usually see positive benefit from these lifts within a week or two. I found that after my own minilift, my face continued to tighten in a lovely, natural way for more than six months afterward. I noticed a constant increase in the "you've never looked more rested" compliments as the months rolled along.

Complications

The complication I most dread after a lift is the loss of a large area of skin from a hematoma. This happens, albeit very rarely, even when a gifted physician using perfect technique does the surgery. Be sure your doctor provides you with a telephone number where he or she can be reached all day every day. Temporary or permanent hair loss, temporary or permanent numbness of the skin, and infection are also possible. Cosmetic surgery is elective; people can live well without it. My whole approach to the well being of my patients is to do the smallest procedure that will yield the highest benefit for the least risk and inconvenience.

The Cost

The classic facelift can cost anywhere between $5,000 and $10,000. Add on a browlift and the price will rise another $1,500 to $3,000. Remember, the deeper and more extensive a face- or browlift, the more costly it will be. Multilevel lifts can easily cost $15,000 or more, a four-lid eyelift can be from $4500 to $6500, and collagen shots are $300 to $400 apiece. What did Lucretia's surgery cost, including face, eyes, neck, new skin, fat transfer? About $12,000.

FREQUENTLY ASKED QUESTIONS

How long do facelifts last?

Let's say your face looks like a clock at midnight, and after a lift we've turned the clock back to nine. The clock, however, doesn't stop ticking and, as soon as the lift is done, you start aging again at the same rate as before. None of these procedures freezes your appearance at a certain age. Unfortunately, we can't stop time. But you will get to midnight later and look better when you get there than you would have without the surgery.

Do you have to shave the hair on my head to do these lifts?

When I do the minilift and minibrow, I never shave the hair. After a minibrow there is sometimes a small amount of temporary hair loss along the stitch line from the shock of moving the skin, but this can almost never be seen, and the hair will start to grow back normally after about a month.

In all my years of practice I have only seen permanent hair loss once, in a heavy smoker who went right back to smoking after surgery. This bare patch didn't show when her hair was styled, and I later did a hair transplant that corrected it.

**Will the minibrow lift give me a perpetually startled,
"deer in the headlights" look?**

This can only happen in a full coronal browlift and not in a
minibrow lift, and it shouldn't happen in any lift at all.

When can I go back to work?

With the minilifts, people can often go back to work in less
than a week, although sometimes two weeks are needed. The
kind of work done is a very important determinant. Heavy lifting and bending are totally forbidden for two weeks after
surgery because they can lead to bleeding under the skin. Working out is prohibited for the same reason.

Chapter 10

THE BODY BEAUTIFUL

LIPOSUCTION, LIPOSCULPTURE, AND LIPOSCULPTION

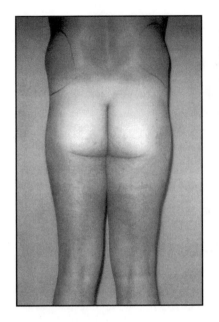
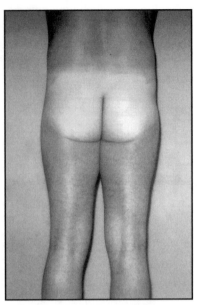
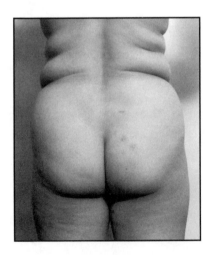
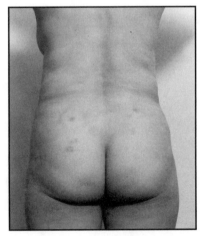

(above) Liposculpture of lovehandles—before and after
(below) Liposculpture of back fat pads (no skin removal)—
before and after
(opposite) Liposculpture of stomach and thighs (no skin removal)—
before and after

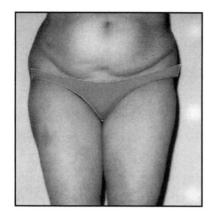 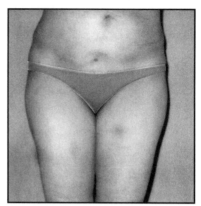

W orking out, dieting, and shaping up are the mantras of the last twenty years, but none of these things can alter our genetic destiny and change the basic body shape we inherited from our parents. If Dad has a spare tire and Mom has ballooning saddlebags, we are very likely to get them as well. Rowing our way across the ocean on our basement machine, being the first to arrive and the last to leave our aerobics class every single day, and putting ourselves on a totally organic, macrobiotic, tofu-enriched, New Age–correct diet will never change that inherited shape. An exercise regimen is good for our overall health, but it will not redirect our genetic path. Although dieting makes us smaller and working out makes us firmer, only liposuction can make us proportional.

In 1984, I first heard that a doctor in Paris had invented a method to remove unwanted bulges from hips, stomachs, saddlebags, heavy knees, and male spare tires *permanently.* It sounded so fantastic that buying the Mayo Clinic for $1 would have been more believable. Nevertheless, I went to Paris to see Dr. Yves

Gerard Illouz at work, I trained by his side on a series of trips, and my career was never the same. The moment I first saw him operate, I knew liposuction was on the level. While in Paris I met men and women he had done the surgery on in years past, and they were among the happiest patients I'd ever seen. To sculpt the human form, to make bodies proportional, to do for people what they could never do for themselves has become one of my most rewarding achievements.

I've inherited many fine gifts from my father's side of the family, but there are two not-so-fine traits I got: one's a gene for baldness, and the other's for having a skinny frame topped with a spare-tire belly. No matter how much I worked out (and I work out *a lot*), those love handles wouldn't go away—until I had them lipoed out in 1984. I love it when women now tell me I have a great body for my age, and I love looking good in jeans or in a bathing suit, much of which is thanks to that lipo work.

One of my patients, Leigh Whitten, says,

> I was a U.S. Gold Medalist in figure skating who always had muscular, large "thunder" thighs, and I know they kept me from achieving my fullest potential in the judging. I was good-looking, in good shape, but I had that pear look anyway. So you could say that ever since I was a little girl who wouldn't wear a skirt above the knees because of my thighs, I've dreamed of having this fixed. Now, I even wear jumpsuits. If only I'd known how much liposuction would contribute to my personal happiness, I'd have done it years ago.

Another great example of terrific liposuction candidates are women who've given birth and, no matter how hard they try, just can't get their old shape back. With lipo, they can reward themselves for their labors, so to speak, with a whole new sexy body and get a big esteem boost to boot.

How It Works

It is generally believed by scientists that, after puberty, the number of fat cells in the body remains the same for life, with weight gain and loss only making these cells larger or smaller. When these cells are removed by liposuction, it is believed that new cells will not take their place. In the fifteen years I've been doing liposuction, I have never seen anyone lose the shape improvement that liposuction gave them. The struggle almost all of us have to maintain an ideal weight is neither harder nor easier after liposuction. If we eat too much after lipo, we'll gain weight exactly as before, but not in the specific bulge areas that made us disproportional in the first place. Weight gain will make us a bigger version of the improved body liposuction gave us.

It was in the 1970s that physicians in France, Switzerland, and Italy simultaneously began working on the solution to the age-old problem of improving the shape of the body. The first attempts by these intrepid doctors were very hard on their patients because they all tried to use rotating, sharp, cutting devices to remove the fat. There were horrendous complications in as many as 30 percent of these patients, including skin loss, infections, and profound denting and dinging. These doctors were great pioneers in their field, but those early years were plagued by gaps in the understanding of how the fat's nerve and blood supply functioned.

Dr. Yves Gerard Illouz of Paris is credited with inventing the modern "blunt method" that made the procedure safe; his work is the foundation of all our understanding of liposuction today. The blunt method employs hollow, blunt rods (*cannulas* in French) to remove the fat. Skeptical ex–New Yorker that I was (and still am), I went to Dr. Illouz's clinic in Paris three times starting in 1984 to learn his techniques and benefit by his enormous experience. On the day I met him, my knees were knocking because I was so nervous. That day I observed him using the cannulas he had designed to remove fat from the hips, saddle-bags, knees, love handles, and stomach of three patients. During the three trips I made to work with him (and a fourth trip I made to work with one of his early collaborators, Dr. Pierre Fournier), I watched many patients have the surgery, and watching the doctors do consultations, I developed a sense of who'd be a good candidate and who wouldn't.

From the doctor's point of view, liposuction is a totally blind procedure, since the small entry points used to introduce the hollow tube under the skin to extract fat are best hidden in natural folds (such as the belly button or the crease of the knee), and because the fat is extracted from a distance. The only way to know the depth of the tube under the skin (or even to know where the tube ends) is to feel, with the hand. Since the vast majority of cosmetic surgery procedures are done under direct visualization, by sight, working by feel isn't natural or intuitive for cosmetic surgeons.

The problem of how to develop a "feel" for liposuction was solved for me by Doctor Illouz. I will never forget the moment when, as he was working, he invited me to put on sterile surgical gloves so that I might actually rest my hands on top of his. After several days of feeling the surgery through his hands, he even let me put my hands in direct contact with the patient's skin so that I could feel it directly. Doctors who learn liposuction at medical conventions, attending lectures and video presentations, don't have an opportunity to learn the touch. Of all the cosmetic surgery procedures I know or have seen, learning the touch of lipo is the most important aspect of becoming great at it.

What I saw in Paris is still the basic way liposuction is performed today. After the skin is cleansed with antiseptic, all areas to be treated are injected with a modified salt solution to both soften the fat and reduce blood loss as it's removed, a technique now referred to as the "tumescent" method. This solution must marinate in the fat for twenty to thirty minutes and, after the wait is over, small incisions are made in the natural creases of the body as close as possible to the area from which the fat will be suctioned. Incisions for the stomach are made in the belly button (or low down in the pubic hair) to hide them, knees are done through the knee creases, and saddlebags through creases at the bottom of the buttock. All these incisions are less than a half inch at most and generally heal well. The cannula (attached to a flexible clear plastic tube that goes directly to the high-powered vacuum machine that gives the procedure its name) is inserted, and the lipo itself proceeds.

As the surgeon works, the hands give the brain completely different information. One directs the procedure, while the other acts as an extractor, moving like a piston. Being a righty I use my right hand to move the tube to and fro, very much like the bow of a violin. The faster I go back and forth the faster the fat comes out of the person, down the tube, and into the collecting bottle. The left hand feels the cannula through the skin and fat by gently lifting up the skin so that the hand goes around it. I call the left hand the "thinking" hand, because by feeling both the tube's location and the thick fat pad actually getting thinner as the fat is extracted, this left hand is telling my brain what it needs to know—the "touch" of lipo.

As the procedure progresses, tunnels under the skin (like Swiss cheese) are made at all different depths of the fat, of different sizes, and going in different directions in order to leave a smooth result without dents, dings, steps, or other irregularities. Areas should always be reduced in a way that makes them harmonious with neighboring areas that are not being done, creating a unified look throughout the body. The body is literally being sculpted, and it's crucial that the surgeon not only have sound technique, but also a real eye for the beauty of the human form.

Liposuction in any form is a fabulous experience for the surgeon performing it since he or she can actually see the body change. While doing a saddlebag, I look at the general shape of the leg so that I remove just the right amount. As I do the hips, I'm looking at the dimension of the waistline, the width of the shoulders, and even the ribs.

One of the sets of photographs in the insert illustrates this point by showing a woman patient in the various stages of a liposuction. Notice that in the middle picture, only one of the saddlebags is gone. Dr. Illouz said that any doctor could make any patient smaller by simply doing liposuction until the collecting bottle was full, but for a true artist the goal was to make the body look as if it had been born with harmonious proportions. This is what I strive for, and his words and the words of all the great teachers I have ever had are always with me.

On my first trip to see Dr. Illouz in Paris, there was a Renoir exhibit at one of the museums. All the women Renoir painted were plump and would be considered heavy, or zaftig, by current styles. The day after I went to the exhibit, I said to Dr. Illouz how fortunate it was that liposuction was evolving in modern times when people liked to be fit and thin, because if it'd been invented at the time Renoir painted, no one would have done it. He smiled patiently and told me to go back to the museum and look again, not at the size (weight) of the women Renoir painted, but at their proportionality and shape. I was amazed the next day when I realized that no matter how large were the women he painted, the bodies were always harmoniously proportioned.

I've visited many museums around the world since and couldn't help but notice that all males and females painted from the most ancient times until the present are generally depicted as having proportional shapes, yet modern studies of human form tend to show that the vast majority of people don't have proportional bodies naturally. Perhaps the human eye innately seeks the beauty of a well-proportioned body that transcends any current notion of correct body weight or size. Liposuction is not a surgery that would be popular only when thin is in, but it is instead a tool for correcting the imbalances and distortions of human form that have bothered people from earliest times.

When the suctioning is finished, small stitches are sewn into the entry points and the body is slipped into a girdle that looks like it came from the 1800s, when women wore "foundation garments," and that reduces swelling and applies compression to define your new body's shape. The girdle stays on for one or two weeks, but you can wear your regular clothes on top of it and get out of the house in one or two days. Most people return to work after four days, so, for example, you could have lipo on a Thursday and be back to work the following Monday. Amazing, isn't it?

Liposuction in a sense is one-dimensional in its ability to help people, but people are three-dimensional. The ideal candidate is, in general, relatively young, not particularly overweight, has good skin tone that is not too loose, and has isolated fat bulges. This leaves out a lot of people, particularly those with loose skin, which is often seen in those who gain and lose weight repeatedly or in women after pregnancy. Lipo for them is a no go because if too much fat is removed from these areas, the skin would loosen even more and become unsightly. Traditional liposuction is additionally unable to improve textural problems like cellulite, the progressive dimpling of the skin that looks like large-curd cottage cheese. (Dr. Illouz used to say that we make new bodies "with the original fabric.") Liposuction was a great technique to add to the repertoire of cosmetic surgery, but we needed more.

Liposculpture

Dr. Luiz Toledo of São Paulo, Brazil, is the great thinker today in liposculpture, and almost everything I use in my liposculpting techniques I learned at his clinic during a series of trips in 1990. This technique takes body sculpting to another dimension: not only are the unwanted bulges removed as in liposuction, but the texture and looseness of the skin are improved.

In liposculpture, the high-powered vacuum machine is replaced by using syringes of various sizes along with longer and thinner cannulas. What happens is that, in the body, there are actually two fat pads in most places, one superficial and one deep. One of Dr. Illouz's key teachings was to do most of the fat removal from the deep and never from the superficial, since if you work too near the surface you will see the outline of the tunnels through the fat, and the skin will undulate, looking like a putt-putt golf course. Trust me; you wouldn't like it.

The use of the syringes and smaller cannulas, however, lets you remove very superficial fat without any telltale hills and dales in the skin. For people like me, this advance was as exciting as getting my first color television set. Because the superficial fat is attached to the skin, you can also scratch the underside of the dermis while suctioning the fat and, in the months after surgery, as the fat pad shrinks, these scratches act as mini-injury points that slowly contract, tightening the skin as well. At the start of this chapter is a visual example of how much a loose stomach tightens without any skin removal, cutting, or need for a tummy tuck with its big scars.

Cellulite is caused by connective tissue cords that surround the superficial fat, and those cords can be broken with a medical instrument that looks like a pickle fork. Reinjecting a bit of the harvested fat will keep the cords from reattaching. The results are not perfect and the skin will not be as smooth as a baby's bottom, but there is real improvement in the dimpling, and the technique is getting better all the time.

Using a cannula attached to a syringe enables the surgeon to "hand fashion" human form in a very delicate way, even actually outlining muscle groups in the stomach and inner thigh to give people an athletic look. So many people work out, run, and do situps, but never have anything to show for their efforts because the well-developed muscles they sweated to get are forever hidden by those inherited fat pads. For the first time, arms can now be tightened and heavy inner thighs can be narrowed, making the legs look longer.

A final advantage of liposculpture is that the harvested fat can be reused in many wonderful ways. This fat can be used to reduce wrinkles of the face, plump up aged wrinkled hands, or firm up and lift a sagging buttock. Most patients at the consultation are so eager to get rid of the fat they've been struggling to reduce their whole lives that, at first, it's hard to convince them that some of it can be put to good use. Many articles about fat reinjection say the fat is rapidly and totally absorbed, but that's not my experience as a doctor, or as a patient. Over the years I've had three fat transfers to improve my own wrinkles and plenty of the filler fat is still there. For most people, 20 to 30 percent of the injected fat will survive for many years if the fat transfer is done with good technique. The rest is harmlessly absorbed by the body. Twenty percent survival doesn't seem all that great until you compare it to injectable collagen, where there is a 100 percent absorption, usually in the first two to six months. I injected some of Geraldo Rivera's fat deep into his forehead on national TV in 1992 (this show was forever memorialized by people such as Johnny Carson, Jay Leno, and Arsenio Hall as the "butt head" show, because the fat I reinjected into Geraldo came from his posterior), and it is still there.

To sum up, liposculpture was the first three-dimensional approach to the body beautiful because it not only reduced disproportional bulges of fat on people, but could both tighten loose skin and even partially smooth out the dings of cellulite. The living fat that is harvested in liposculpture can be very useful for softening wrinkles and even filling in body hollows such as the low point between the hips and saddlebags seen in many women. This great advance has made the body beautiful available to a lot more people. Remember the narrow list of people who were good candidates for liposuction? Liposculpture can be performed on people who are a lot older, have loose skin, and are bothered by cellulite.

LIPOSCULPTION

Liposculption is a term that you will never see in a medical book; it's a term I made up to describe my modification of machine liposuction combined with the use of the best techniques of liposculpture and, most important, the mindset of the surgeon.

For four years I sculpted whole bodies with only a syringe and let my liposuction machine get dusty. I then realized that for very large inherited bulges (particularly saddlebags and hips), the machine could produce more dramatic results because of its greater power. To avoid leaving those skin depressions, I used lower power settings and had cannulas made that were longer and thinner than normal, and coated with Teflon, reducing the need for so many large entry points.

The mindset of the surgeon, however, is what really sets liposculption apart. Though some people just want to reduce a single area of their body (which is how traditional lipo doctors are trained), the vast majority of patients have several areas that need treating simultaneously. Just as no two men or women are shaped alike, no single technique can optimally sculpt all people with good results. For example, think of the stomach: some stomachs have tight skin (suggesting the modified machine approach), while others are very loose (needing a hand approach that uses syringes to tighten the skin). Even if the stomach skin is tight, I will use small syringes to outline the muscles for an athletic look after using the machine to remove the bulk of fat. A surgeon with the liposculption mindset will use every technique, instrument, and method at his or her disposal to give each individual patient the best body possible. It has taken me many years to learn to harmoniously combine the best of the past and present in my work, and my quest to find even better ways to give you the body you've always wanted will never stop.

ULTRASOUND LIPOSUCTION

Ultrasound is the latest lipo development, and I went to Paris in 1994 to see if it was safe and a genuine improvement in technique. In this procedure, after the tumescent liquid is injected to prepare the fat, an ultrasonic probe is used to break down the fat cells and emulsify them, making them more amenable to suction. Proponents of the method say that contouring is better because the work for the surgeon is easier and faster, and one can remove very large volumes of fat from obese people. Opponents say ultrasound lipo costs a lot more because the machines, which are not used in any other areas of the cosmetic surgeon's practice, cost the doctors around $50,000. Additionally, there've been cases of severe burns to the skin and fat (because of the heat generated by the sound waves), loss of large areas of skin, large dents in the skin, and even several cases of severe blood loss. On top of all that, the technique is just not yet refined enough to do the key feathering needed to ensure a seamless transition between the affected areas and the neighboring areas so that no steps or dropoffs are seen. This means surgeons still have to do liposuction or liposculpture at these transition areas.

What do I really think of ultrasound lipo? I don't really know yet, but I think some of the hullabaloo misses a very important point. At best, this technique, if refined and made safer, could in the future replace some of the modified machine liposuction I do now. But no technique like this can be used for the body sculpting that I love: it can't tighten loose skin, delicately outline muscles, or improve cellulite. It is like turning back the clock twenty years on all our terrific liposculpture advances.

The Preparation

Prior to surgery all patients are required to have a blood test to make sure there are no underlying abnormalities, especially an inability to clot normally or anemia. In older people or people with heart disease or lung disease, a physical examination, electrocardiogram, or even a chest X-ray may be required. People with high blood pressure, diabetes, or even those with heart disease may be able to have liposuction safely, if their illnesses are under good control and their family doctor approves. Aspirin and aspirin-containing compounds as well as all alcoholic beverages are to be stopped at least two weeks prior to surgery because they greatly increase bleeding and bruising. Patients are urged to come to the office the day of surgery in comfortable, loose-fitting clothes, such as a sweatsuit that will easily fit over the postop girdle.

The Procedure

I have almost never known a patient who didn't have a case of "buyer's regret" the morning of surgery. The fact that patients actually get to the office without turning the car around is something I don't take for granted.

The first thing that happens is the bill gets paid. Most cosmetic surgeons require full payment the morning of surgery, while some require full payment a week in advance.

The next step is usually to sign a consent form, designed by a battery of lawyers, that is always frightening. It is very important that the potential complications written in the consent form are the same ones that were mentioned in the consultation; otherwise, you are not legally informed when signing. After reviewing and signing the form, you'll change into a paper gown to be photographed. Superb quality preop photos are key to evaluating the results as the months go by.

Lipo procedures can take as short as forty-five minutes or as long as four hours, if several areas are being sculpted. I have had patients have liposuction on the midface, neck, midback, breast pads, stomach, back, arms, hips, saddlebags, inner thighs, knees, and ankles all at the same time. This is not too much surgery to have at once, and in fact, if all these areas need adjusting, it will save you much time, convenience, and money to have them all done together.

If you're having one area done, such as the stomach, you can be made comfortable with just local anesthesia (Lidocaine) and a little IV sedation to relax you. If you are having many areas done at the same time, a regional or general anesthesia may be required. Some patients just want to be "knocked out," a phrase I hear very often before starting. There are no hard and fast rules. Anesthesiologists are among the most individualistic of all doctors: no two work in exactly the same way and their recipes are equally personal.

Afterward

After the surgery the patient spends several hours in a recovery area where vital signs are monitored in preparation for going home. Don't even think about hailing a taxi or taking a bus; you won't be up to it. A loved one or a friend should be on call, and someone should sleep in your home and be available to you for one or two nights.

Most surgeons give patients a postop sheet reminding them to take it easy for a few days and not make any important personal or business decisions (the effects of anesthesia after large procedures may not fully wear off for up to a week). The sheet will also specifically mention signs of infection and any other symptoms of side effects or complications. If you develop a high fever, see bleeding from the incision sites, or experience any of the other warning signs mentioned in the sheet, don't wait—call right away, any hour of the day or night. Small problems in medicine that can easily be corrected if acted on quickly can become much more difficult in the space of just a few hours.

The vast majory of postlipo patients only need some Tylenol, but extensive work can really hurt the next day. The pain is not sharp but is instead a deep soreness very much like a sports injury. The worst of it lasts one or two days and can be reduced by the generous use of strong pain pills. After several days you are still stiff and sore but getting more comfortable all the time. People often go out for walks the next day and even begin light workouts at the end of a week.

Jayne remembers that "the recovery included a lot of soreness, like an intense lower-body workout with weights; the pain lasted about a week. The real results don't come for three to six months later, but, boy, was it absolutely worth it. The only thing I could think was, why didn't I do this years earlier? Now I really have the look that I deserve for working out like I do. I'm more confident, especially in a swimsuit; it really does change your whole attitude."

If you are recovering from lipo, listen to your body. If you're doing an exercise that doesn't feel good, your body is telling you it is just too soon. If you persist, you will not harm the lipo, but you will prolong the stiffness and soreness.

The girdle usually comes off after one or two weeks of shaping and molding you. Many patients tell me they keep the girdle on longer, under their clothes, because it feels good and gives them an idea of what their future, improved shape will be.

After a single-area lipo, most people are back to work in one or two days. When you have the "works," plan on missing about a week. Your body will be red, white, and blue all over afterward, and the skin will usually remain heavily bruised for about two weeks. Stitches usually come out in two weeks, and then the real waiting begins.

The Results

Very few cosmetic surgery procedures show immediate benefits, and this is especially true of liposuction. In the first few months, the skin will feel doughy or woody from the deep swelling, and in a few people, the swelling will make your body look larger for a few weeks, making you think you had a lipoaddition instead of a suction. You are also likely to see temporary dents and dings in the skin, but these will smooth out in the months afterward. During the first two months after surgery even the sturdiest patients are more than a little worried and even disappointed. After all the presurgery worry, the pain after surgery, and the cost, patients generally want concrete results as soon as possible.

In general, the best benefit will be seen after four to six months. Each passing month, as the contour and proportionality of the body improves, your decision to take the plunge will be validated again and again.

Complications

An infection after lipo would worry me more than with other types of cosmetic surgery because infection could rapidly spread through the tunnels in the fat. Fortunately, this has never happened to one of my patients, but it can happen, even when lipo is done with perfect technique. Because of this, I give everyone an antibiotic regimen during surgery and for one week after.

Permanent grooves, waves, and dings can occur. The question I have asked myself over the years is: can this complication be eliminated by enough experience and perfect technique? But even Doctor Illouz himself says no. When I met him he had already done more than three thousand procedures, and he said that no matter the skill of the surgeon, such waves and dings still occurred from time-to-time in predisposed patients.

Two days before writing this sentence, I did lipo on a man who had a spare tire. At the very beginning, as I was making my first tunnels in his love handles, I immediately saw a groove in the skin, which is not supposed to happen, so I stopped what I was doing and switched to a thinner cannula, totally getting rid of the groove by working around it and injecting a bit of fat from the other side to elevate it.

The point is that some patients are more "sculptable" than others, just as some mediums are more sculptable than others. Some people have skin and fat that imprints in such a way that a small fat removal would lead to dings if the surgeon didn't catch it at the beginning and switch to another technique. You need to make sure that your doctor gets ding-free results most of the time and, most important, that he or she is handy at correcting it if there is a problem.

Finally, some lipo patients have actually had heart attacks, fluid in the lungs from overexuberant IV fluid replacement, penetration of internal organs by the cannula, and some have even died. That said, Dr. Illouz has never had these dreadful things happen to his patients, and neither have I. In fact, lipo is among the safest of cosmetic surgical procedures. The risk of these complication is so low that I have had fat removed from my own love handles (yes, I am looking for the body beautiful, too) and have performed lipo on thousands of patients in perfect safety.

The Cost

Most liposuction surgeons charge by the area of the body. In my practice the fee would be the same if you did the stomach only, the hips only, or the knees only. As is the case with facelifts, a discount is usually given if multiple areas are worked on at one

time. A surgeon might charge $3,500 each for hips or saddle-
bags, but $5,500 if both are done on the same day. This discount
stems from the fact that so much of the cost of cosmetic surgery
is in overhead and throwaway supplies like sterile drapes, syringes, and suture material.

Costs are variable, with the stomach, for example, going for
between $2,000 and $5,000. Some surgeons charge extra for doing larger areas, while experienced surgeons specializing in liposuction generally charge more. Doctors in large cities and
other high cost-of-living areas are usually more expensive than
those in the suburbs.

You can check costs by asking several local doctors who are
considered experienced and specialized in the technique. Patients often feel uncomfortable negotiating a price for surgery,
but in fact, though physicians operate on people while vets
work on animals, there is more horse trading in negotiating a
cosmetic surgery price than most patients imagine.

FREQUENTLY ASKED QUESTIONS

Can the fat come back?

This is by far the number-one question, and another way of
asking if the results are permanent. People have more than 10
billion fat cells, and according to current scientific thinking, the
ones that are removed cannot regenerate. In my fifteen-year experience no patient has ever come back and said the love handles or thick knees ever came back. I think of myself as creating
a new pattern for your body with liposuction. The new pattern
should hold up for the rest of your life.

What happens if I gain weight later?

This is the key question. Even if a large liposuction permanently rids your body of hundreds of millions of fat cells or

more, the remaining fat cells are just as eager to take up any extra calories you throw their way as they were before. Some people think that liposuction replaces dieting or working out to reduce weight or even allows a person to eat as much as they want. If that were true, it would even be more popular than it is today.

Maintaining weight afterward is not any easier than before, but the difference is that you will show the weight now in areas from which fat cells were not removed. If you gain weight you will keep your improved shape, but you can easily become a larger, obese version of that better shape.

Is male fat different from female fat?

Usually fat in men is firmer and more fibrous than fat in females, and many surgeons use different instruments when doing liposuction on men.

What about the male "beer belly"?

Before I started doing lipo, I thought that many of the men you see on the beach with huge bellies would be great candidates for it, but I was wrong. Most men with enormous waistlines have virtually no fat in the skin itself. Instead the fat is deep in the body cavity surrounding organs such as the stomach and intestines where it cannot be readily reached.

Will pregnancy void the benefits of liposuction?

Many younger women who want liposuction haven't had babies yet and they worry that a pregnancy will diminish the contour improvement they get from the surgery. I have never seen this happen. It is certainly true that, when pregnant, the shape and weight of a woman's body changes dramatically, but after the baby is born and the body returns to its former shape, the full benefit of liposuction also returns.

How old is too old to have liposuction?

I have done successful and safe liposuction on men and women who were more than eighty years old, but it's rare. Patients who come to me in consultation have told me that doctors they have consulted with have said that forty is the maximum age for having the surgery. In my opinion, it is hard to set an absolute cut-off age since I see forty-year-old men and women with eighty-year-old bodies, and forty-year-old men and women with twenty-year-old bodies. Each person must be evaluated individually.

Chapter 11

THE BREASTS

A SOUTH AMERICAN PERSPECTIVE

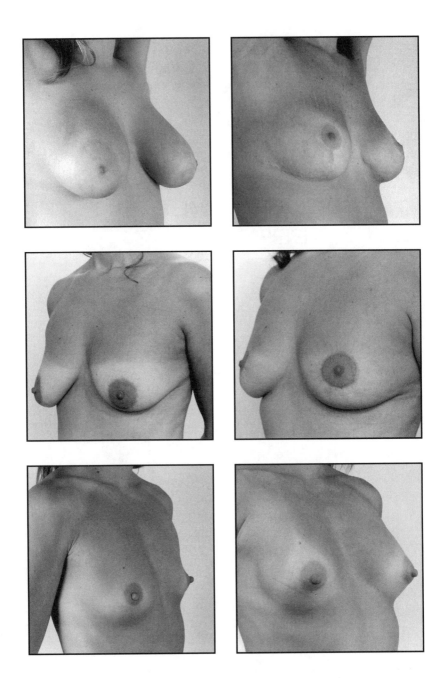

(above) Breast Reduction and Mastopexy with the inverted
T-incision—before and one year after
(middle) Periareolar Mastopexy—before and one year after
(below) Breast Augmentation with a 150 cc prosthesis—before and one
year after

We need no poetry to explain the importance of breasts as part of a woman's body. Beauty and function, curves and volume, everything seems so simple, yet so precise. Textures of softness to enchant and to feed. We could go on forever. The subject is fascinating.

When nature is kind, and beauty helps, everything is wonderful. But not everyone is blessed with the perfect pair of breasts, and plastic surgery can help as a last resort. There is no way to improve breast shape other than surgically.

The beauty ideal varies according to several factors: type of body, age, race, and yes, even geography—there are basic differences in preferences regarding the shape and size of breasts from country to country.

AUTHOR'S NOTE: I wrote this chapter after interviewing colleagues in Brazil who specialize in breast surgery, and it represents a Brazilian or South American point of view.

Patterns of Beauty

The preference in Brazil is for the whole breast to fill one cupped hand. Even if it's a big hand, the average American woman usually prefers bigger breasts, not to mention the Texas women who tend to like them even a little bigger and the many male admirers who want them beyond imagining.

When a Brazilian woman wants a breast implant, the average size she chooses is 150 cc, and rarely will she want it larger than 200 cc. Surgeons in the United States, meanwhile, use a minimum size of 200 cc and commonly go larger than that, with an average American prosthesis (implant) of between 250 and 300 cc. Otherwise, they think, why bother?

Brazilian women prefer their volume in the buttock, rather than in the chest. Obviously there are cultural, ethnic, psychological, and aesthetic reasons for these differences of opinion, something not even Freud would have dared try to explain. But it is a fact.

Once the prosthesis of desired size has been chosen, the actual shape of the breast doesn't change much: a slight concave curve running down from the shoulder and ending at the tip of the nipple, returning to the chest in a convex curve. The breast should be firm, as if about to explode, but it should also be as soft as the baby's mouth that reaches for it.

The poetry of the perfect breast is disrupted when nature is unkind. One can be born with small breasts, breasts that are uneven in size, breasts that become too big, too flaccid, or too low, not to mention the ravages of breast cancer, which can affect one in every ten women.

There can often be strong psychological undertows for a woman unhappy with her breasts, for whatever reason, and this cannot be overlooked. Postsurgery reports show that patients have an improved body image, a decrease in self-consciousness, and a heightened self-confidence.

Usually, middle-aged women who seek breast reduction complain that their heavy breasts cause pain in the neck, shoulder, and back regions and leave dents on their shoulders caused by bra straps. Younger women often refer to more psychological and cosmetic reasons for seeking breast reductions.

There are basically five types of problems. The breast is either:

- too small (needs to be augmented);
- too big (needs to be reduced);
- too fallen (needs to be raised);
- too small and too fallen (needs to be augmented and raised); or
- too big and too fallen (needs to be reduced and raised).

Plastic Surgery Techniques

Over the past four hundred years, at least, there have been reports of surgeons trying to solve the aesthetic problems related to the breast, but it was only in the beginning of the twentieth century, with the improvements in anesthesia, that surgeons could effectively change its shape.

The dilemma of the plastic surgeon has always been to find the right balance between the shape of the breast and the size of the scar. Several techniques have been developed and perfected to obtain the best possible shape with the least visible scar, while maintaining the function of the breast—function meaning not only breast feeding but also sexual stimulation.

The problem of obtaining the best shape with the smallest scar is common to all aspects of body contouring, and the main solution to this came with the invention of liposuction in the late 1970s. Since then, we've been able to remodel the shape of the body and the face using only small incisions.

Hypertrophy is a medical term meaning an increase in size. It is not unusual for breasts, especially in adolescence, to increase in volume and become hypertrophic, usually due to an excess of fatty tissue, and it was specifically with this type of patient in mind that we started using liposculpture to reduce the volume. This excess weight can cause back problems, problems with posture, and psychological problems related to self-image.

Today we can reduce the breasts, by one or two bra cup sizes, using the syringe liposculpture technique, a relatively simple surgery performed under local anesthesia on an outpatient basis. This procedure can enhance the shape and size of the breast using only very small incisions. The breast will still undergo changes in the future with pregnancies, lactation (nursing), and the passing of time when a more extensive procedure might be indicated.

The same technique can be used to treat adolescent boys who sometimes suffer from gynecomastia, the development of small breasts during puberty. A combination of liposculpture and a small incision to remove the gland can solve this and avoid the obvious psychological problems that could follow this condition.

Breast Augmentation

The classic technique for breast augmentation (breast aug, for short) was developed in the 1960s. It is a straightforward technique that consists of placing an implant, a bag of silicone gel or a saltwater solution known as saline, under the breast through a small incision. This technique is used to augment a small breast, to balance a difference in size, to correct a reduction in breast volume after pregnancy or weight loss, and, of course, following breast cancer surgery as a reconstructive technique.

Saline gel implants have been used safely for breast augmentation over the past thirty years. The implant itself, however, can provoke the formation of a fibrous connective tissue capsule around the implant surface. This is a normal reaction by the body, and though it should not be obvious or felt, in some cases (about 20 percent), this fibrous tissue undergoes a contracture, a hardening of the implant where it can clearly be felt as an unnatural lump, which can be solved by replacing the implant.

In the 1980s there was a great advancement with the development of the textured capsule breast prosthesis, which dropped the contracture rate to a mere 1 percent. But, sometime in the early 1990s, an American television program stated that there was insufficient information to prove the safety of silicone gel–filled breast implants, leading the U.S. Food and Drug Administration (FDA) to rule that the new gel-filled implants could only be placed in women who were participating in scientific studies, until the implant's safety was proven. Today, the only type of breast implant approved by the FDA without restriction in the United States is the saline-filled one, but this could change at any time and you should consult your doctor. Because the saline implant does not have the soft texture of the gel, it makes the breast firmer. Many of my professional colleagues believe the silicone gel–filled breast implant is the best available, but because they are currently banned here, many American patients fly to other countries to have their breast work done.

Some women complain that after a breast augmentation the nipple becomes more sensitive, less sensitive, or numb. These symptoms usually disappear between the second and sixth postoperative months but might be permanent depending on the technique that was used.

Breast implants can sometimes break or leak as a result of trauma or from the compression of the breast on the implant. With a saline solution implant, the escaped liquid is reabsorbed by the body in a few hours. If a silicone gel implant leaks, the body can form a fibrous capsule around the implant. If the breaking is due to a trauma, this can provoke migration of the gel to other areas, usually the underarm, where the body will form some scar tissue around the gel to contain it. This requires a second operation to clean up the area and replace the implant.

Some women have reported joint pain or swelling, fever, fatigue, or breast pain. So far, it has not been proven that these symptoms are related to silicone breast implants, but the FDA has requested further studies. The fact that the implant manufacturers have already agreed to pay billions to patients without conclusive scientific evidence should make any person very hesitant to ever have silicone implants even if the FDA allows them again.

Breast augmentation is one of the procedures with the highest degree of patient satisfaction in plastic surgery, and although you might not have any of these complications, it is always wise to discuss the possibility with your doctor during the consultation.

The Procedure

The anesthesia used can be general, regional, or local. I prefer a combination of local with IV sedation, the so-called "twilight anesthesia." The anesthesiologist controls your vital signs and will put you to sleep with light hypnotic drugs. The breast is injected with local anesthesia and the process is totally painless. There are three different incisions through which the prosthesis can be inserted. The choice of which incision to use should be made in a consultation between patient and surgeon.

The submammary fold incision, placed in the horizontal fold under the breast, is the most commonly used and gives immediate access to the area. Through a one- to two-inch incision, depending on the size of the implant, the surgeon will create a "pocket," an empty space under the breast, cauterize the blood vessels, and insert the prosthesis. The incision is closed and the dressings put in place. The submammary scar is usually hidden by the weight of the breast. The procedure, both sides, takes less than an hour.

The areolar incision can be periareolar (around the areola) or transareolar (across it). The periareolar incision is made on the border of the color difference between the normal breast skin and the darker skin of the areola and, because of this, is usually well hidden. The transareolar is also well hidden although some surgeons tend to avoid this technique because the nipple and areola have to be divided and then sutured together again, and some doctors worry that nipple sensation might be affected. Surgeons who use this technique say it doesn't interfere with the milk ducts or nipple sensation. Of these two methods, most surgeons prefer the periareolar.

The third style of incision is in the armpit, or axilla. This is usually preferred by women who do not to want any scars on their breasts whatsoever. The incision can only be seen when the arms are raised. It is a little trickier placing an implant through the armpit incision, and once the pocket under the breast is dissected, it will be necessary to cauterize any bleeding vessels with the help of an endoscope (a device for looking under the skin) before closing the incision.

Once the incision placement is chosen, it is time to choose where to place the implant, either between the breast gland and the pectoral muscle or under the pectoral muscle. The anatomy of the chest follows this sequence: skin, fat, gland, pectoral muscle, rib cage. It is believed that the implant placed between the gland and the pectoral muscle will give a more natural shape but will show a possible contracture more easily. The implant placed between the muscle and the rib cage has less chance of showing any possible capsular contracture but will tend to sit higher on the chest because of the contraction of the pectoral muscle. All of these decisions should be made between the patient and surgeon once the pros and cons of each have been explained and discussed.

A medical support bra must be worn for a month to keep the implants in place. The dressings should be changed daily for seven to ten days, after which time the stitches are usually removed. Movement of the arms should be restricted to a minimum in the first two weeks following surgery. Driving and the carrying of heavy weights should be delayed until the tissues can move without bleeding, usually around the third postoperative week. Any kind of sports activity or sunbathing is forbidden for at least a month, but after that a new life with more confidence and self-esteem begins. When body and mind are in harmony, we live with a more positive attitude and we get what we want from life.

Risks

All types of surgery have risks but breast augmentation is a relatively simple procedure with minimal risks. When capsular contracture occurs, removal of the scar tissue or removal or replacement of the implant is required. Swelling and some pain can occur following the operation and, to a certain degree, should be expected. If there is excessive bleeding after the surgery, however, this will have to be controlled and another operation might be needed to remove any coagulated blood. Cases of infection around an implant are minimal and will usually occur within a week after surgery. In rare cases, the implant is removed and, after the infection clears, a new implant can be inserted. This process can take several months.

Breast Reduction

Today there are probably as many techniques as there are surgeons. Well, not exactly, but it is true that almost every surgeon has a slightly different method of doing a traditional technique. Today there are three main types of incisions used for breast reduction: the inverted T incision, the L incision, and the periareolar incision. The inverted T is the most widely used. Several techniques use this approach because through this incision it is possible to maintain the integrity of the breast, its function, and also improve its shape. The final position of the inverted T incision goes around the areola, from the areola to the submammary fold, and then horizontally along the submammary fold, forming the shape of an inverted T.

The internal treatment of the gland can vary a lot according to the surgeon. First, the areola and nipple are dissected and elevated to their new position, the excess gland is removed in a keel shape, and the breast is mounted and sutured into place. The external stitches will be removed between the tenth and fourteenth days, and a support bra must be worn for the first postoperative month. Some surgeons will insert drains to keep blood from collecting, and these would be removed on the fifth to seventh postoperative day.

The L-shaped incision is a modification of the inverted T. Few surgeons have the expertise to perform this technique, but the ones who do show beautiful results and are strong advocates of the procedure.

The third type is the periareolar technique, a T incision that leaves a scar only around the areola. It is a very difficult technique with very specific indications, but it is the ideal approach for small deformities. But when used on large breasts, a flattening effect is produced, again illustrating the battle between the ideal shape of the breast versus the size of the scar. With this technique there is a very small scar, but the shape can suffer.

Mastopexy

Mastopexy is the surgery to elevate the fallen breast and any of the three incisions mentioned above may be used. Instead of removing gland, only the excess skin is removed and the breast is molded to its original position. This technique is designed for women who are happy with the size of their breasts and who look great with their bras on, but whose skin is too flaccid to hold the breasts in place without support. Mastopexy postoperative care is the same as that for breast reduction but usually has a faster healing time because the changes are more superficial.

Breast Augmentation and Mastopexy

The combination of breast augmentation and mastopexy can also be accomplished through either of the three basic incisions. The excess skin is removed and the implant is placed to achieve the desired size. This combination, however, should be carefully carried out, because if the skin envelope is too tight the scars will tend to stretch.

Scarring

Long-term scar complications include hypertrophy and keloid formation. A hypertrophic scar is caused when the suture line enlarges and stretches, usually after the second month. A keloid is a benign skin tumor that causes an unsightly but harmless thickening of the scar. Keloids defy logic. It is not unusual to see a patient with a long scar who develops keloids in only a few areas of the scar, with no plausible explanation. Keloids are usually genetic, but not always. Thus, having a keloid scar on one part of the body doesn't necessarily mean the person will have keloids on the breast scars and so cannot undergo breast surgery. Keloids can be treated either by a superficial type of radiotherapy called betatherapy, with the injection of diluted amounts of cortisone, or with external compression with a silicone gel dressing.

Breast Reduction and Mastopexy

The main area of caution during this surgery is when the breasts are very large. The elevation of the areola to its new position has to be carried out very carefully so as to maintain its blood supply. If the blood supply is jeopardized in any way skin or nerve sensibility may be effected.

Sensitivity

A decrease in nipple sensation can be expected in the first two to six months after surgery, depending on the technique utilized, although some women report an increase in sensitivity. After a few months, however, the breast's sensation should return to normal, with the muscles of the areola contracting and arousing the nipple.

The scar healing process takes longer. There are three stages, the first ending around the fifteenth day when the stitches are removed; the scar at this time will usually look good and be almost imperceptible. The second period reaches its peak at the third postoperative month when the scar becomes redder and more noticeable. The third period ends only at the eighteenth postoperative month, when one can say that the scarring process has been completed and there will be no further changes. With age, scars tend to become more imperceptible.

Different Breasts

There are cases where the breasts are different and uneven. Obviously no one has perfectly identical breasts; there is always a slight difference, and this is all part of the balance of beauty. However, in some women one breast develops significantly more than the other, and the surgeon will have to choose the right technique to correct this problem. In some cases it is not always possible to operate on one side only and it may be necessary to alter both breasts to obtain good symmetry.

The Cost

Like all surgery, there is a range of price depending on the procedure, the surgeon, the health facilities required, and the region where you live. In general, the range is $7,500 to $11,000, broken down into a doctor's fee of $3,000 to $6,000; $2,000 to $4,000 for the hospital and assistants; and $1,500 for the breast prostheses.

FREQUENTLY ASKED QUESTIONS:
REDUCTION AND MASTOPLEXY

Will the sensation be preserved on my breasts?

The nipples and areolas are not detached from the underlying tissues, so you can have preservation of sensation. Ability to breast feed is normally unaffected, but this depends on other factors and can't be guaranteed.

How will my scars heal?

There are different variations in the incisions for breast reduction, according to the size and shape of each person's breast. Sometimes it is possible to leave a scar only around the areola, sometimes there's a vertical scar. The more traditional inverted T scar, with its horizontal part underneath the breast, is the most common.

When can I go back to my normal activities?

Usually it is possible to return to work after from one to two weeks, depending on the occupation. There's usually a wait of two weeks to drive an automatic car and, if there are no bruises left, a month before beginning mild exercise.

How long before I can have sex?

As any sexual activity can involve an increase in blood pressure as well as physical exercise, it should be avoided for at least one week. Ask your surgeon about your specific case. *Gentle* is the watchword here.

How long will I have to wear a bra?

Your doctor should prescribe how long the use of dressings and a molding bra will be necessary; usually it is around one month.

FREQUENTLY ASKED QUESTIONS: AUGMENTATION

When can I go back to my normal activities?

From five days to a week, depending what you do; violent arm movements should be avoided for three to four weeks.

How long before I can have sex?

Any sexual activity should be avoided for at least one week. After that your doctor will decide, keeping in mind that the area of the breasts should be treated with extreme gentleness.

What type of implants will be used?

In 1992, the Food and Drug Administration decided that silicone gel–filled implants can't be generally used for cosmetic breast augmentation, so saline-filled implants are used instead. This is a very controversial issue, and things are expected to change as soon as we have new scientific data on the safety of the gel-filled implants.

Where will the scars be?

Insertion of saline-filled implants requires only a one-inch incision that can be made underneath the breast. Other implants may require a two-inch incision. The incision can also be made around the areola or in the axilla (within the armpit).

What are the risks of contraction?

After a breast implant surgery a fibrous scar capsule is formed as part of the healing process. Sometimes this capsule can be too thick and too tight and therefore might compress the prosthesis. This can happen in different degrees. When the fibrous capsule is too large, it may have to be removed and the implant replaced.

How long will the implants last?

Breast implants are not expected to last forever and a periodic mammogram is necessary to evaluate the integrity of the implant. If there is a rupture, or if the implant breaks for any reason, say during an accident, it will be necessary to remove the implant and replace it.

Will the implants hide a possible breast cancer?

Today we use MRI (magnetic resonance imaging) and ultrasound to detect very small tumors even in the presence of breast implants. Your plastic surgeon should be able to advise you on a good specialist with experience in performing MRIs on breast implant patients.

Chapter 12

✳

THE NOSE

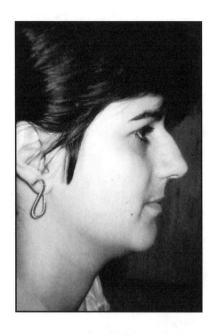
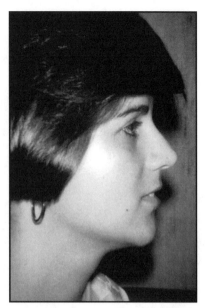
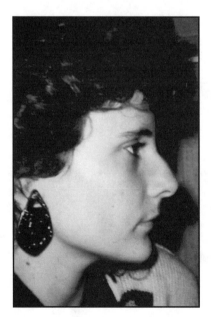
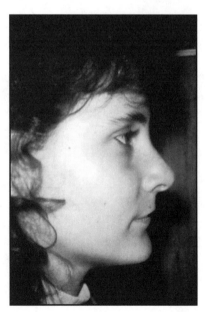

Rhinoplasty procedures—before and after

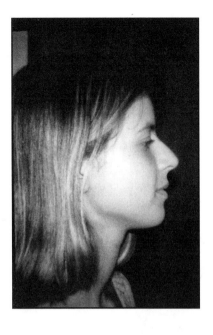
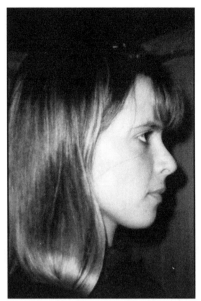
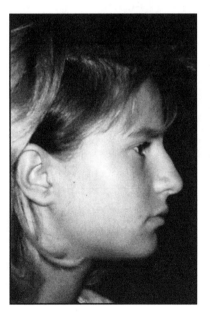
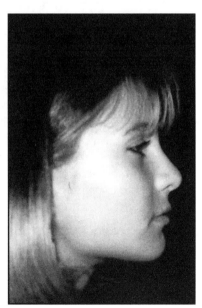

BY DR. ALBERTO CESAR HODARA,
DR. REMO FARINA JR., AND
DR. DEBORA LESSA NORA, MEMBERS,
BRAZILIAN AESTHETIC PLASTIC
SURGERY SOCIETY

All of these doctors teach at the
University Medical School in Porto Alegre, Brazil,
and have one of the largest practices in Brazil.
More important, they are my great teachers!

In spite of what is commonly believed, rarely do patients approach cosmetic surgeons wanting to be more attractive than the norm. Instead, they come to us to improve something about their appearance that keeps them from looking their best. The patient believes some part of his or her body is too small, too big, too thin, too broad, too long, too short, or too crooked and wants to change this in order to achieve harmony. In this chapter we try to help the reader understand what is available in rhinoplasty—the aesthetic surgery of the nose.

The nose is among the most important features of the face in determining symmetry, balance, and visual personality. It is at the end of puberty that the nose takes its final shape; its aesthetic effect, for better or worse, manifests itself at that time. The nose constitutes three distinct structures: the bony base at the top; the long section made of cartilage; and an outer covering of skin. Dissatisfaction with any of these elements can cause a person to consider rhinoplasty. There could be a bump or a growth on the bony or cartilage areas; there could be an overdeveloped growth of cartilage, or an overdeveloped nasal partition making the nose look too long. The surgeon must respect the size and proportions that will allow the nose to be integrated naturally into the overall scheme of the face.

How to Choose a Surgeon

Do some research, become educated. Talk to doctors you know and trust, find friends and acquaintances who've shared the same aesthetic problem and were pleased with the results of their surgery, do research in libraries and magazines. Rhinoplasty is the kind of surgery that must be done right the first time out, since making corrections after the fact is often very difficult and sometimes impossible.

The Consultation

The consultation day is perhaps the most important day in rhinoplasty as this is when you must describe to your surgeon exactly what it is about your nose that you don't like. Too often, a patient and doctor talk with each other without paying attention to what the other is really trying to say (in Brazil this is called deaf talking), with the surgeon not listening to the patient's main complaint and expectations and the patient not listening to the surgeon's explanation regarding the procedure's limitations. You can avoid this deaf talking by listening carefully to everything your surgeon says and making sure you understand each other. More than is the case with most procedures, it is crucial for the surgeon to make sure that the patient has reasonable expectations and a realistic view of what it is possible to achieve. Someone who is depressed or obsessed with his or her nose is not a good candidate for surgery and should be discouraged from having it. Someone who has had one or several procedures done before, all of which had unsatisfactory technical or emotional outcomes, should not be operated on again.

Consultation is also the time for the doctor to inform you when the procedure can be scheduled, what you need to do beforehand, how long the procedure will take, the kind of anesthesia involved, the length of the recovery, and what you can expect afterward in terms of healing. Practically any patient over the age of seventeen can undergo rhinoplasty since by that age the nose is fully grown and its final shape can be completely planned. If you have a chronic illness (such as diabetes, hypertension, or mild heart disease) that is well managed, and your medication is being taken properly, there is no reason not to go forward. The doctor must be told about any drugs you are taking, whether sleeping pills, painkillers, or anything else. Anyone suffering from a respiratory infection (whether it's the common cold, flu, or pneumonia) or any other severe infection must be cured before rhinoplasty can be considered.

Finally, the nose will be carefully examined; the widths of the center and the bottom of the nose (the nostrils) are important considerations. From the profile, any unwanted hump near the top of the nose, the projection of the tip of the nose, and the length from where the nostril meets the skin of the inner cheek will be examined. Pictures will be taken from several angles to provide a detailed record to guide the surgeon's hand. Here's another chance for you to make sure your surgeon knows exactly the result you're looking for.

Several consultations are sometimes useful before making a decision. Many patients are justifiably worried that they'll wind up with a nose too small or turned up, a nose that says "nose job." It is easy to explain to the patient that today's techniques allow the achievement of a result very close to what is anticipated.

The Procedure

You'll stop eating at least eight hours before surgery and will arrive at the doctor's office wearing no makeup or facial lotions. The kind of anesthesia chosen depends on the patient's physical condition, on the doctor's evaluation, and on the patient's preferences; it can be local or general. The surgery is usually done in an outpatient clinic. Patients generally go home the same day or the next day. It is best to arrive in comfortable, loose-fitting clothes. After the surgery, you must have someone ready to take you home and someone should stay with you overnight.

The Technique

Today's rhinoplasty has been greatly advanced to provide the best outcome possible. We can take actual measurements of the face and look for a perfect harmony among its parts. This is important because, in some cases, it is the other parts of the face that need improvement. For example, a very thin face combined with low projection of the cheekbones and dental arches may make you look like you have a big nose, but what you in fact need to correct is the chin or the dental structures. Rhinoplasty will not accomplish what you think it will in a case where other facial features are out of proportion. We also have modern techniques that enable us to diminish or enlarge the nose vault, to straighten it, to elevate its tip or make the tip more pointed, to narrow the nose bones, and even to redraw the contour of the nostrils themselves.

In most of the procedures, the surgeon can operate on both the cartilage and bone through short, invisible incisions on the inside of the nostrils: a hump in the profile of the nose can be eliminated, a low or high tip of the nose corrected, the nose narrowed, a deviated septum corrected. If the bottom of the nose, by the nostrils, is too wide, a small amount of the nostril skin can be removed to narrow it. In this case, there is a small skin incision, but it can be well hidden in the natural crease where the nostril meets the skin. To narrow a broad nose, external incisions must sometimes be made at the lateral fold of the nostrils, but these become virtually invisible in a few months (or in a few days, thanks to makeup).

Afterward

Immediately after surgery, the patient will have a swollen face and mild bruises around the eyes or on the eyelids, and the swelling and brusing can last from one to three weeks. It's very useful during the recovery period to keep the head up, even for sleeping, as this will shorten the recovery time. If the patient doesn't care much about the edema (swelling), the bruises, or the surgical dressing, some activity can be resumed after forty-eight hours.

The inside of the nose is usually packed with gauze to stop bleeding, and this packing is left in place for one to four days. A splint of plastic is placed on top of the nose for seven to twenty-one days to keep the bones of the nose together and offer additional protection until the early healing period is over. The stitches inside the nostrils are self-absorbing, so it's not necessary to remove them. Exercise and other hard physical activities should be avoided for at least two months. The final result won't be seen until the sixth postop month, when the healing process is completed.

Complications

Infection is uncommon because the nose has such a tremendously rich supply of blood, but it's common to take antibiotics after surgery to reduce the risk further. Bruising, however, is very common and sometimes blood can accumulate under the skin (hematoma). Postop nosebleeds can be stopped by applying pressure or repacking the nose. Because the blood supply to the nose is great, severe hemorrhage after surgery can sometimes, albeit rarely, occur. The doctor can stop the hemorrhage by locating the source and cauterizing it. If the surgeon has removed too much bone or cartilage during a rhinoplasty, there may be a loss of structural support for the nose, or even the loss of skin, which can lead to scarring.

If the result of the surgery is unsatisfactory, more surgery can be done when the nose has completely healed, after six to twelve months. Such surgery is called secondary rhinoplasty and occurs in 10 to 30 percent of cases. Secondary rhinoplasty is very much more complicated than first-time rhinoplasty because scarring or restoring structural support for an overdone nose is more complicated.

The Costs

Rhinoplasty will run $2,500 to $5,000, depending on the extent of the surgery and where you live.

FREQUENTLY ASKED QUESTIONS
BY DR. JAMES ROMANO

Doctor Romano is a Johns Hopkins–trained board-
certified plastic surgeon. He practices in San Francisco
and is a colleague and good friend.

What in general is done during rhinoplasty?

Rhinoplasty procedures are done either for reduction or augmentation. In reduction, the nasal bones are often made more
narrow, the top of the nasal bone and cartilage are made flatter,
and the tip is reduced and refined by removing excess cartilage.
In augmentation rhinoplasty, cartilage from the septum inside
the nose is borrowed and placed on a low or sloping top of the
nose and often used as a support to raise up a drooping tip. Not
every patient will need their "bones broken."

Where are the incisions placed for rhinoplasty?

There are two generic types of rhinoplasty techniques. In the
closed rhinoplasty, all incisions are placed inside the nostrils. In
the open rhinoplasty, there are incisions inside the nostrils and
a small incision that crosses the bottom center column of the
nose.

What is the commonest complication of rhinoplasty and how often does it happen?

Poor cosmetic result, although rare, can happen in about 5
percent of cases, and this is often related to the underlying
anatomy and the complexity of the surgery.

Do I need to be completely asleep for the surgery?

Rhinoplasty can be very safely performed under general anesthesia or "twilight" local anesthesia. Most doctors use an anesthesiologist in both situations. The difference may depend only on patient preference or on any underlying medical conditions.

I don't want to look like I've had a "nose job."
Can rhinoplasty be done to look natural?

This should be every surgeon's goal. The results of rhinoplasty depend on careful assessment of the patient's perspectives, goals, and nasal anatomy by a doctor who clearly sees these things and can provide a natural, balanced, and graceful result. It is most important to determine if your doctor shares your aesthetic perspective. Rhinoplasty should not change your natural look.

When can I return to my normal activity and exercise?

After rhinoplasty, a splint is placed on the nose. Once the splint is removed, one can return to normal daily activity, including light exercise, though there should be no bending or stooping or heavy lifting for several weeks. Contact sports and vigorous activities should be delayed for about six weeks.

To what degree are swelling and bruising present,
and how long do they last?

There will be a variable amount of swelling and bruising depending on the extent of the surgery. The swelling is greatly diminished after the first to third week, but the last small amount will resolve slowly over the next six months. Bruising usually lasts about seven to ten days, but not every patient gets "raccoon eyes." Most patients can return to social activities by the end of the first week.

When will I see my final result?

When the packing is removed after one week, 90 percent of the cosmetic result is immediately apparent. The final appearance will be seen when the six-month period of complete healing has ended.

Do I need packing, and when is it removed?

Doctors are finding that fewer and fewer patients really need packing. If packing is used, it is removed two to seven days after surgery, and this is not painful.

Will rhinoplasty affect my breathing?

If a patient undergoes a significant reduction in the size of the nose, then breathing problems may result if not anticipated and planned for at the time of surgery. Specific maneuvers at the time of rhinoplasty should improve breathing in patients with a history of difficulty and should not ever make breathing worse.

Can rhinoplasty be revised or redone if I do not like the result?

Yes, secondary rhinoplasty can be performed. Surgeons try to avoid this since your best result is often obtained at the initial surgery. If there is some opportunity to "touch-up" or make a rhinoplasty result better, it is often delayed for at least six months to one year after surgery to allow for all the swelling to completely subside.

✳

SUMMING UP

FROM CYBERSPACE
TO INNER LIFE

I was twenty-eight years old when I decided to become a dermatologist, and thirty-five when I began to specialize in aesthetic surgery. At those times, I knew relatively little about what these jobs would be like. I have changed a lot as a person in the twenty-five years since, but looking back at my career now, I couldn't be happier with the decisions I have made.

From as long ago as I can remember, my parents taught me that serving others was the most important thing you could do with your life. Though I can admire anyone who makes good widgets, when your job is to make human beings feel better about themselves and genuinely improve their lives, you feel that your own life really has purpose and meaning.

I know that plenty of doctors (and especially the HMOs) run an assembly line type of medical practice, and probably I'd be more successful business-wise if I'd done that too. But I've always thought of myself as my patients' employee and I consider myself fortunate that they trust me enough to place their welfare in my hands. All my surgery patients get my unlisted home num-

ber, and I'm always there anytime they need me, day or night—
but this hasn't been a one-way street. With a divorce and the
deaths of loved ones over the years, I've had plenty of my own
personal problems, and I've drawn incredible strength and support from my patients through their love and respect. Just to see
the happiness that the surgery I perform gives them, and to see
their own lives improve because of it, has sustained me through
some of the most difficult times of my life.

When I began creating a World Wide Web page for my cosmetic surgery practice nearly three years ago (www.look-
young.com), I was breaking new ground, providing valuable
information on how cosmetic surgery works for browsers from
anywhere in the world, and communicating with people in need
via e-mail. I made sure the site was not just a boring bulletin
board describing a long list of procedures; I filled it with anima-
tion, virtual reality, morphing, before-and-after photos, and
even audio tapes from shows I'd been on, such as *Geraldo*. To this
day, the most popular pages at the site are two animations that
show a heavy neck turning thin and a lower body becoming
shapely.

There are many people who want to know about cosmetic
surgery, but they are so shy that even calling a doctor's office
anonymously to get general information would be too much for
them. These people can browse the site repeatedly, learn a great
deal about the procedures they are interested in, and no one will
ever know. The site has been designed so that a great deal of information can be learned quickly, but it also has enough depth
that hours and hours can be spent browsing for more detailed
information. Many people I have met in consultation have told
me that they would never have felt comfortable calling the office or coming in person if they had not been able to first
browse the site in the comfort and privacy of their homes.

People who have been injured in accidents or have been born
with defects such as cleft palates will e-mail me for help in getting referrals where they live. Some have confided in me the sor-

row and helplessness they feel when a child or loved one has been burned or had an injury that has dramatically changed the lives of everyone in the family.

Most e-mail I receive contains requests for information about particular procedures—will they solve the concerns of the e-mailer, how much do they cost, how much time will be missed from work, and what are the risks of the surgery. I often ask these people to send photos for me and my staff to evaluate. Sending a short letter and photos is often just the icebreaker needed to get someone to seriously think about having cosmetic surgery.

As you must know by now, I am tremendously excited about all the medical breakthroughs in my field that have helped me improve my work. But I'm just as excited about bringing aesthetic surgery "out of the closet" and more into the mainstream of everyday life. As I've said over and over again in this book, cosmetic surgery is no longer only for the rich or the elite; it's for anyone who wants to match physical appearance with inner life.

PLASTIC SURGERY AS THE SEARCH FOR BEAUTY AND WELL-BEING

BY DR. IVO PITANGUY

Doctor Pitanguy, who practices in Rio de Janeiro,
Brazil, is considered the godfather of plastic surgery.
The inventor of modern breast surgery,
Doctor Pitanguy is a true living legend.

The search for inner harmony as a means for reaching personal well-being is an important issue that universalizes beauty. In essence, this is the main goal of every aesthetic surgical procedure. Excluding extreme cases, most patients approach a plastic surgeon wishing to improve their appearance to achieve better integration with their social group. Acceptance in the community is generally the main motivation of the patient, and once this is obtained, a greater self-esteem is almost always achieved as well.

The ideal of beauty is always individual, a subjective standard that depends on extrinsic factors (ethnic group, religion, geographic situation) and intrinsic factors (temperament, sensibility, culture). Each race and culture has its own concept of beauty that varies according to different periods of time. Identification with his or her group defines the standard of beauty and behavior of the individual. When people lived restricted in their tribes, this group identity was more easily preserved since geographical distances kept groups isolated from one another. Nowadays, issues regarding the body and its physical representations, together with the influence of the advertising industry, have so changed aesthetic ideals that many times they invade patterns established by religion, race, or age groups. Boundaries established by social barriers and aesthetic standards have been lost.

Beauty lies deeper than the surface of form. Although beauty is easily recognized, defining it is a complex task, and it becomes necessary to reflect on its different and fundamental concepts. Beauty has recently been defined by theories that consider art as its fundamental expression. "An object cannot be beautiful if it can give pleasure to nobody," said Santayana. "When our senses find what they crave—then perception is pleasure."

These concepts help us to better understand this science-art that is plastic surgery, since, in the last analysis, it allows for the patient's identification with his or her search for beauty. In fact, this search has been expressing itself through the ages and through different populations in an extensive variety of artistic manifestations. However, it now becomes necessary to examine the role of plastic surgery in this search for beauty, for in its inherent limitations lie the factors for patient dissatisfaction.

A few famous plastic surgeons have pronounced themselves on this subject, and their statements may help us understand the aim of our specialty: "We restore, repair, and make whole those parts of the face—not so much that they may delight the eye but that they may buoy up the spirit and help the mind of the afflicted" (Gaspare Tagliacozzi, 1597, medieval surgeon, professor at the University of Bologna, and first to write about psychology and cosmetic surgery). Prominent German surgeon Gustave Aufricht has said, "The justification of any operation is the good for the patient." I myself have said: "If we consider beauty to be the ultimate fulfillment, and that its external manifestations are different in each particular ethnic group, what we surgeons seek, then, is to decrease the deformity rather than re-create beauty."

The plastic surgeon should evaluate the desires of the patient within his or her own aesthetic standards, taking into account the idealization the patient may be creating of the final result. A balance between the patient's self-image and the one he or she idealizes is necessary for the best result. Analysis of the equilibrium between body image and the possible result offered by the surgical technique is a task that requires a keen sense of empathy and sensibility on the part of the surgeon. In this way, the eye of the surgeon looks for the role the sense of beauty plays in the aesthetic demands of his patient. These demands will influence the subjective inner identity: the image the patient has of him- or herself.

The surgeon, a slave to form and anatomy, frequently becomes frustrated when manipulating the human body, since a more noble material has yet to be created; he removes and adds, having to follow the laws of the body. This limitation—what the surgeon can offer, considering the structures and tissues of each individual—must be explained to the patient in detail. A perfect and ideal result should not be assured, since this can never be guaranteed. New technological equipment that allows the surgeon to create an image for the patient tends to bring a perilous precedent, since it suggests that this idealized outcome will be the final result the patient can expect.

The aim of a facial rejuvenation operation is not to achieve eternal youth, because the surgeon should not be seen as a new Mephistopheles handing Faust a magic potion, as in Goethe's epic poem. The purpose of surgery for the aging face is to allow the individual to live the experience of commuting between youth and old age in an active and harmonic manner. Aesthetic facial surgery has witnessed enormous progress over the last twenty years, and is sometimes described as a relatively complex procedure. Consequently, the expectations of both the patient and the surgeon have increased considerably. The basic principles that have stood the test of time should always be remembered. The surgeon must be knowledgeable in details of surgical technique and its variations so as to attain the best result for each case. Facial anatomy should be examined carefully for an individualized diagnosis. It should be stressed that the patient seeking an aesthetic facial procedure is often anxious about the possibility of an unnatural result. Distortion in anatomical landmarks and permanent visible scars are a constant worry because they announce to the world that the patient has had surgery. The bond created between the patient and surgeon will be broken if there are any signs that surgery has been performed.

Plastic surgery is therefore a means that may help a patient find his or her inner self, recovering a dynamic equilibrium with the outer world. Many times, success in this medical specialty is based on the deep relationship that develops between the doctor and his patient, and so it is indispensable for the plastic surgeon to determine if the needs and hopes of the individual are compatible with what the surgical procedure can offer. In plastic surgery as in other surgical specialties, the patient presents not only a physical complaint but also strong emotional issues. It is fundamental that each case undergo a careful selection and an assessment of the real benefits that an indicated procedure may achieve.

All physician-patient relationships must be based on trust and honesty. The patient must express his or her wishes, and at the same time, the surgeon must try to know the personality of the patient and the corresponding expectations. This dynamic exchange culminates in a final diagnosis and treatment proposal, when the patient is informed of the real possibilities and possible untoward results of the procedure. As Aufricht commented: "The plastic surgeon who deals with these patients knows that they are not submitting to surgery out of pure vanity. Vanity would be the desire to exceed others. In the vast majority, what patients really seek is just the opposite. They wish to pass unnoticed, freeing themselves of certain unattractive characteristics."

The surgeon also has the responsibility of emphasizing to the patient that any surgical procedure must be approached with the same seriousness as any other type of surgery. Patients who undergo aesthetic surgery are commonly anxious for a satisfactory final result and many times do not realize the complications of the procedure. In order that risks inherent to any surgery be minimized, the surgeon must assure the patient that a complete preoperative investigation will be done as a routine and that all necessary resources will be available in case of any unforeseen occurrences. On the other hand, the postoperative period is usually a moment of physical and psychological recovery, in which the patient's evaluation of the result may be influenced by subjective issues that should be taken into consideration by the surgeon. Personal conflicts, the influence of third parties, a search for perfection, or secret motives previously kept hidden (sometimes unconsciously) may cause a degree of dissatisfaction that must be promptly resolved.

✴

GLOSSARY

Abdominoplasty: The tummy tuck corrects stretched skin in the belly usually caused by repeated weight gain and loss or pregnancy; loose skin is removed, and the underlying muscles tightened.

Augmentation mammoplasty: The enlargement of the breast using an artificial implant filled either with saline (saltwater) or silicon (only outside the United States).

Blepharoplasty: The eyelid lift that removes the extra skin and fat that cause a droopy or fatigued expression.

Botox: A naturally occuring chemical derived from bacteria that is injected into the muscles of the forehead to temporarily relax them and erase wrinkles caused by their use.

Chemical peel: A face peel, using phenol or trichloroacetic acid, that removes wrinkles and age spots.

Collagen: A protein derived from cow skin and injected into wrinkles and lines to temporarily plump them up.

Dermabrasion: A surgery that smooths out scars on the face by removing the skin's outer layer.

Liposuction: Removal of the fat lying just under the skin through the use of a cannula and vacuum.

Liposculpture: Replaces the vacuum with a syringe.

Ultrasound liposuction: Uses ultrasound to break down the fat before it is removed.

Mastopexy: A breast lift that removes the extra skin and repositions the nipple in a higher position after pregnancy and nursing or gravity have pulled the breast down.

Mentoplasty: The augmentation of the chin with an artificial implant.

Otoplasty: The repair of the ear; most commonly used to make a protuberant ear lie more flatly against the head.

Reduction Mammoplasty: Reducing the size of the breast by removing extra skin and fat.

Rhinoplasty: Surgery of the bone and cartilage to improve the appearance of the nose.

Rhytidectomy: A facelift. Skin is repositioned in order to counter the aging effects of gravity.

BIBLIOGRAPHY

Adams, Gerald R. "The Effects of Physical Attractiveness on the Social-ization Process." *Psychological Aspects of Facial Form.* Monograph 11: Craniofacial Growth Series, Center for Human Growth and Develop-ment. Ann Arbor: University of Michigan, 1981.

Berscheid, Ellen. "An Overview of the Psychological Effects of Physical Attractiveness." *Psychological Aspects of Facial Form.* Monograph 11: Craniofacial Growth Series, Center for Human Growth and Develop-ment. Ann Arbor: University of Michigan, 1981.

Colman, David. "Old-Fashioned Vitamin C as the Hot New Beautifier." *The New York Times,* 21 September 1997.

George, Leslie. "Improving on Nature." *Self,* September 1997.

Georgiade, Gregory S., Ronald Riefkohl, and L. Scott Levin. *Plastic, Max-illofacial and Reconstructive Surgery,* 3d ed. Baltimore: Williams & Wilkins, 1997.

Ivy, J. E., Z. P. Lorenc, and S. J. Aston. "Is There a Difference? A Prospec-tive Study Comparing Lateral and Standard SMAS Facelifts with Ex-tended SMAS and Composite Rhytidectomies." *Plastic Reconstructive Surgery* 98:1135, 1996.

Nash, Joyce D. *What Your Doctor Can't Tell You About Cosmetic Surgery.* Oakland, Calif.: New Harbinger, 1995.

Downsizing of America. New York: Times Books, 1996.

Webster, Richard R. C. "Introduction: The Growth of Surgical Expertise and Organizations in Dermatology." P. xvii in *Principles of Dermatologic Plastic Surgery,* Marwali Harahap. Baypoint, CA: PMA Publishing Corp., 1988.

Yoho, Robert A., and Judy Brandy-Yoho. *A New Body in One Day.* Studio City, Calif.: First House Press, 1997.

INDEX